The best value beauty book ever

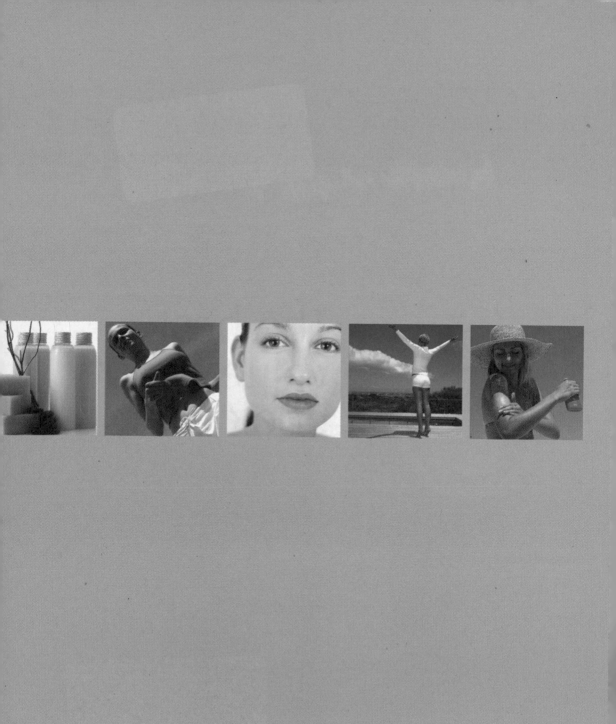

THE BEST VALUE

Beauty

BOOK EVER

Linda Bird & Eve Cameron

infiniteideas

Careful now

We want you to look your beautiful best but we're not your Fairy Godmother. You're a grown up now so it's up to you to take responsibility for your own appearance. The tips in here need to be combined with effort on your part in order to work so if at first you don't succeed have a think about whether it was your approach rather than our advice that was at fault, and then have another go. We know there's a gorgeous creature lurking inside so get out there and start turning heads.

Although the contents of this book were checked at the time of going to press, the World Wide Web is constantly changing. This means the publisher and author cannot guarantee the contents of any of the websites mentioned in the book.

Acknowledgements

Infinite Ideas would like to thank the following authors for their contributions to this book: Linda Bird, Eve Cameron, Kate Cook, Peter Cross, Helena Frith Powell, Lisa Helmanis, Clive Hopwood, Lynn Huggins-Cooper, Cherry Maslen, Lizzie O'Prey, Marcelle Perks, Steve Shipside and Elisabeth Wilson.

Copyright © The Infinite Ideas Company Limited, 2007

The right of the contributors to be identified as the authors of this book has been asserted in accordance with the Copyright, Designs and Patents act 1988.

First published in 2007 by
The Infinite Ideas Company Limited
36 St Giles
Oxford
OX1 3LD
United Kingdom
www.infideas.com

A CIP catalogue record for this book is available from the British Library

ISBN 13: 978-1-904902-85-0
ISBN 10: 1-904902-85-5

Brand and product names are trademarks or registered trademarks of their respective owners.

Text design and typeset by Baseline Arts Ltd, Oxford
Cover design by Cylinder
Printed in India

Brilliant ideas

Brilliant features

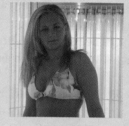

Each chapter of this book is designed to provide you with an inspirational idea that you can read quickly and put into practice straight away.

Throughout you'll find three features that will help you to get right to the heart of the idea:

- *Here's an idea for you* Give it a go – right here, right now – and get an idea of how well you're doing so far.

- *Defining ideas* Words of wisdom from masters and mistresses of the art, plus some interesting hangers-on.

- *How did it go?* If at first you do succeed try to hide your amazement. If, on the other hand, you don't this is where you'll find a Q and A that highlights common problems and how to get over them.

Introduction

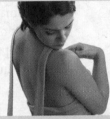

Beauty is a difficult concept to define. It can mean different things to different people, but chances are that at some point in our lives we've all wished we could be more beautiful. How far we choose to pursue that goal is up to us – for some it will just mean finding the perfect shade of lipstick, while others may feel the only way to achieve the looks they want is through surgery. However far you want to go in the quest to be gorgeous we hope you will find some new, exciting and inspirational tips here.

No doubt you will have spent many years leafing through magazines and books for the best ideas and forked out large amounts of your hard-earned cash on clothing, beauty products and gym memberships to boost your looks. Our editors have consulted dozens of authors to bring you the very best ideas on looking and staying beautiful so that now you need look no further than this book for beauty secrets to last you from your twenties to your nineties.

Our experts agree that one of the most important factors in looking beautiful is self-confidence – the way you present yourself to the world can do a lot to hide all your little imperfections. However, you may find that a few simple tricks will be important to you in giving you that self confidence. This book is full of sensible diet tips, clever clothing ideas, artful make-up methods and insights into which products, exercises and techniques work best for top to toe loveliness.

Don't feel you need to try all the tips in order. This book has been designed so that you can dip into it anywhere, any time. If you have a particular problem area – untamable hair, dimply thighs, so-so skin – then turn straight to the relevant idea to sort it out. Other ideas will give you more general advice for all over beauty. Above all we hope you enjoy reading the book. Beauty is simple really – sleep well, eat well, keep an eye on your bad habits (you know what they are) and above all enjoy life.

Look great in photos

Stars and photographers alike know all the tricks. Adopt these clever postures and easy make-up techniques and the camera *will* lie when you want it to.

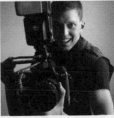

Sticking your tongue into the roof of your mouth will make your lower facial muscles contract and tighten that wobbly double-chin patch. Try it in front of a mirror. Ingenious, isn't it?

Camera-shy or woefully unphotogenic people should commit this kind of tip to memory. Knowing how to show off your most beautiful features will also equip you for those horrifying times when someone feels compelled to 'capture the moment'.

If you watch models and celebrities carefully at red-carpet events, you'll notice that they'll strike a carefully calculated pose as the paparazzi gather. The result? A smaller waist, longer legs, more sculptured cheekbones.

So, next time you have to face your public, try some of the following tricks picked up from the stars and the photographers.

Here's an idea for you...

Maximise your lips. To pout beautifully, turn to the camera and say 'Wogan'. Bizarre, I know, but glamour models swear by it.

- To look your slimmest try standing with one foot slightly in front of the other and gently pivot on your feet so that your body, including your shoulders, is at a slight angle. Putting your hands on your hips can make your waist look instantly smaller.

- If you're sitting down, lean forward and rest your elbows on your knees. That way you'll disguise wobbly thighs.

- Look lively. Greta Garbo *froideur* isn't always the most flattering attitude to adopt in snaps. In fact, some professional portrait photographers insist the best pictures are always taken when the subject is looking animated and chipper. That way the subject's personality is captured. You can still engineer your 'best side' in front of the camera.

- Practise in front of the mirror. Perfect a pose you're happy with so you can strike it the moment the camera comes out.

- Brighten up. Dark colours can often be slimming to wear but black can drain the colour from the face, so choose brighter colours for your top half to bring out the best in your skin tone.

- Beware of brightly patterned clothes, as they can swamp you and detract from your face.

- Dark circles or bags under your eyes? Try lifting your chin to avoid shadows falling on your face.

- Smile. Forget looking moody, as everyone looks more attractive when they're looking happy. Plus a lovely smile really does take the focus away from the bits you're less happy with.

- Poker straight hair can pull your face down. Putting your hair up can soften your features and draw attention to your smile.

- Get the photographer to take more than one photo! The more you have taken, the more likely it is you'll be captured from a flattering angle.

'With charm you've got to get up close to see it; style slaps you in the face.'
JOHN COOPER CLARKE, poet and comedian

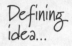
Defining idea...

MAKE-UP TRICKS

You'd be forgiven for thinking that slapping on gallons of foundation and concealer over spots and blemishes will create alabaster skin and hence wonderful photographs you'd be proud to display. Forget it. Overdo the slap and you'll look like a waxwork or, worse, a cross-dresser. Be subtle instead.

- Apply a light foundation only where necessary, such as to the sides of your nose or over spots.
- To avoid a shiny face, stick to matt-formula make-up for your blemishes and only use creamy, reflective concealers for your eyes.
- Flatter your best features. Apply blush over the apple part of your cheeks, sneak a couple of extra false lashes on your eyelids and slick on some glossy lipstick. Don't forget the golden rule of make-up though: never overplay the eyes *and* the lips. Choose between them before you open that make-up bag.
- Ask for a minute or two before the camera clicks so you can touch up and dab a bit of powder over any shiny bits. Who cares if you seem vain? There are few things as insidious as unflattering photos of yourself in someone else's hands.

How did it go?

Q   I have a rather sizeable nose that always looks huge in photos. How can I make it look smaller?

A   You need to gently 'direct' the photographer here. Try to steer him upwards, as taking the picture from an angle above you, looking down, will minimise a big nose and make your eyes look bigger.

Q   I always blink in photos. Is there anything I can do to avoid this?

A   A mistimed blink is guaranteed to make you look drunk or simple. Make it a rule never to look directly at the flash so that you won't blink at the crucial moment. Instead, try focusing on the photographer's head or just above the camera.

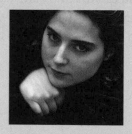 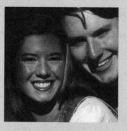

Suck it out: the surgical route to fat loss

An alternative to dieting or the icing on the cake when you've lost weight and need a boost? It's not without risks, so here's what you need to know about cosmetic surgery.

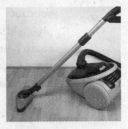

If you don't like your long toes, you can get them shortened. You can swap an 'outie' belly button for an 'innie'. You can even buy J Lo's bottom for yourself.

Cosmetic surgery has come a long way. It is now possible to sculpt away that excess fat. The downside is that it's expensive, it isn't always successful and it might not make you any happier. Surgery is not a good alternative to eating less and being active, which is the safe and sensible approach to weight control. Personally, I do feel that surgery is a last resort, but if you have lost lots of weight and the fat loss has left you with loose rolls of skin, a tummy tuck might give you a confidence boost. The most important thing is to do lots of research, ask questions and find the best possible surgeon.

Here's an idea for you... **Try an instant image change with a haircut. Layers can make your face look slimmer as can highlights. For men, a short, sharp haircut can make you look more George Clooney than Billy Bunter. Great hair works wonders.**

Any surgery carries risks, such as infections, bleeding and reactions to anaesthetic. It's also important to see several surgeons before committing yourself to a procedure and ask them plenty of questions, including the following:

■ How often have you performed the procedure?

■ What kind of anaesthetic is used and who will administer it?

■ How long will the procedure take and how long will the results last?

■ Where will the incisions be and what level of scarring might I be left with?

■ What's the recovery time?

■ Can I see 'before and after' pictures and testimonials from other patients?

WHAT SURGERY IS ON OFFER?

One option for fat removal is liposuction, where a narrow metal tube is inserted into the fatty area via an incision in your skin. The surgeon moves the tube back and forth and sucks out the fat with a vacuum pump, leaving the nerves and blood vessels intact. There are variations in techniques, but that's the general idea. There is a maximum amount of fat that can be removed from an area, so you might not be able to sculpt off as much as you like. It also doesn't affect cellulite (the lumpy, dimply bane of many women's lives) and can leave skin loose. Following the procedure, your skin usually retracts and is bruised and uncomfortable. Healing can take a long time, with lumpiness and swelling taking up to six months to disappear. It's definitely not for the faint-hearted. Neither is a tummy tuck (abdominoplasty). With this procedure, excess skin and fat can be removed and muscles tightened. There are mini, standard and extended versions. All leave a scar, from a low one at the level of the pubic hair to one that extends around to the back. Are you feeling faint at this point? Me too, but let me tell you about a couple of new developments. The latest high-tech techniques include LipoSelection by Vaser, which uses advanced ultrasound technology to separate out the fatty tissue from the rest before it is removed. This is claimed to be more precise, gentler and less painful, with a quicker recovery time. There is also the lower body lift, which pulls up all your slack skin around the hips, thighs and stomach. It is claimed to smooth out cellulite, flattening lumpy 'orange-peel' skin. You can also get arm and breast lifts, and just in case your hands don't match your newly slim and lifted body, there is now plenty that can be done, from getting rid of bulging veins to plumping up saggy hand skin with your very own recycled bottom fat!

Excuse me, I must go and lie down as I'm feeling rather queasy.

'I was going to have cosmetic surgery until I noticed that the doctor's office was full of portraits by Picasso.'
RITA RUDNER

Defining idea...

How did it go?

Q   How much do these sorts of operations cost?

A   Prices depend on individual surgeons and hospitals, and the specific techniques used. However, the cost of a tummy tuck and liposuction would probably pay for gym membership, a personal trainer, a nutritionist and goodness knows what else for at least a year.

Q   How do I find a surgeon?

A   As well as seeking out personal recommendations, check that they are members of a professional body such as The British Association of Aesthetic Plastic Surgeons (BAAPS). New BAAPS members, for example, have to be recommended by two others who are aware of their ability, skills and knowledge.

Q   Is there such a thing as a toe job?

A   Yes. It involves making little incisions, cutting a bit of bone out, then reattaching the tendon. Result? Prettier toes.

3

Feet first

Feet generally don't get a second thought till summer, by which time you really have your work cut out for you. Instead, attend to them daily.

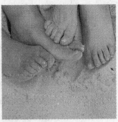

Paying attention to your feet can actually boost your health and well-being, as well as stop people wincing at the sight of them.

Feet get a real beating as apparently we average between about 4,000 and 5,000 steps a day. Most of us spend a lot of our life rushing around in ill-fitting shoes, too, which can cause problems from blisters to corns, as well as exacerbate bunions, back pain and posture problems.

There's a Sarah Jessica Parker in all of us; the only thing separating most women and a serious Manolo habit is cashflow. Women seem genetically programmed to gravitate towards absurdly impractical shoes, but choosing the right shoe for the job can help minimise damage to the foot. When shopping for shoes, try to think first about heavy-duty wear. What will you be doing in those shoes? Walking to work? Rushing around shopping?

Here's an idea for you...

Stimulate acupressure points on your feet. Stiff neck? Gently walk your thumb and fingers across the ball of your foot below your toes then around the base of your big toe. Aching back? Slowly walk your thumb down the inner edge of your foot following the bones along the arch.

Specialists recommend we choose a low-heeled shoe (no higher than 4 cm) for everyday wear, with a rounded toe. We're also advised not to wear shoes for consecutive days because it takes them about 24 hours to dry out thoroughly; and sweaty shoes cause smelly feet and fungal infections.

Wear high heels for a special occasion, by all means, but live in them and you'll damage your feet and cause postural problems. Moreover, they can shorten your calf muscles and make them look stocky.

Wearing tight shoes can also cause bunions, curvatures in the toes and swollen, tender joints. It's worth giving your shoe wardrobe a serious rethink, because wearing tight shoes can make the problem worse. A chiropodist can help you limit further damage by recommending shoes with a straight inside edge, which should prevent excessive pressure on the joint. Also, protective pads can be worn to ease pressure on the joints and shoe alterations or orthotics (special insoles) can help the feet function more effectively. In severe cases, surgery may be necessary.

Regular foot maintenance makes sense and few treatments will make you feel more enlivened than a pedicure or a session with a chiropodist, so budget for a treatment once every three months. The rest of the time:

- Regularly remove hard skin with a pumice stone.
- Trim your toenails with proper nail clippers, cutting straight across and not down at the corners, which can cause ingrown nails.
- Get into the habit of washing your feet each night with warm soapy water, but don't soak them for too long or too often in water that's too hot or you'll destroy the natural oils.
- Stretch your feet and exercise your muscles by making big circles with your feet – clockwise and anticlockwise – and repeat four or five times each.
- Make sure you dry your feet thoroughly, especially between the toes. Smother moisturising cream all over your foot, avoiding the area between the toes, and then apply some foot powder.
- Treat your feet to a regular, soothing foot massage. You can either buy specialist foot products for this, use your favourite body cream or try essential aromatherapy oils diluted in carrier oil.

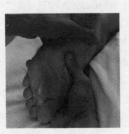
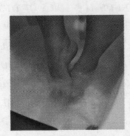

'If high heels were so wonderful, men would be wearing them.'
SUE GRAFTON, writer

Defining idea...

How did it go?

Q   What can I do to tackle the cracked skin on the heels and balls of my feet?

A   *First, try smoothing the area. Use an emery board or pumice to gently rub away the hard bits and then rub in a rich moisturising cream to soften the skin, such as an aqueous cream or E45.*

Q   What can I do to make my feet smell sweeter?

A   *Change your shoes every day and invest in some good foot products. Peppermint-imbued ones are deliciously cooling and refreshing and foot deodorants (even underarm deodorants) can keep your feet feeling and smelling fresh. Choose socks made from natural fibres, preferably cotton, and change them every day. Wherever possible wear well-fitting shoes or sandals that allow air to circulate. Use an anti-fungal powder and spray between the toes.*

Q   What's the best way to get rid of a verruca?

A   *Verrucas are warts usually found on the soles of the feet that usually start out as a tiny pink area with black dots and later become dark brown with a rough crumbly surface. They're caused by a contagious papillomavirus that thrives in damp conditions such as showers, bathrooms and swimming pools. Nice. If the verruca doesn't hurt and isn't getting any bigger, leave well alone. Sometimes covering it with a plaster can cure it. Otherwise, try a gel or ointment from the chemist. If the verruca is painful or getting larger see a chiropodist, who may remove it surgically. Prevention is best, so wash your feet regularly and avoid walking barefoot in communal changing rooms (wear flip-flops or verruca socks).*

12

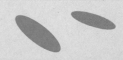

4

Work it!

This is the idea you need when you have to be smart and sassy at 8 a.m. and gorgeous and sexy at 8 p.m. and there is no time to go home in between.

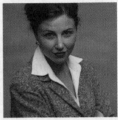

You can't quite believe it's happened. The man of your dreams (and we're talking fairly graphic dreams) has finally asked you out on a date.

Great news. The bad news is that you have a hugely important presentation that day, followed by a client lunch and then a data training session all afternoon. There is no time to go home and freshen up between work and play.

Don't panic. The first thing to do is to start your preparation early. The night before go to bed early, having had a long bath, done your nails, waxed your legs, plucked your eyebrows and so forth. Get into bed wearing a moisturising mask (my favourites are the really thick and creamy ones), don't take it off, but leave it on all night – believe me it's worth the messy pillowcase in the morning.

Here's an idea for you...

Take another pair of shoes to the office to change into for the evening. There's nothing quite as refreshing as taking off shoes you have been running around in all day.

Next morning, have a shower, wash your hair and prepare yourself as you normally would for a day at work. The key is in what you take with you to work. I am guessing you will have at least an hour between leaving work and the date. This time needs to be used to give you that 'just left the bathroom' look and feel. To achieve this you will have to bring to the office make-up remover, face moisturiser, toothbrush, hairbrush, scent, deodorant, new underwear, tights/stockings and a change of clothes. Some little extras could include a product that promises to brighten up your face like a beauty flash balm – most make-up companies do one (but be sure to apply make-up straight away afterwards or it flakes).

Once you have finished your high-powered day, you lock yourself in the ladies' loo. If the one at the office isn't very nice then be bold: walk to the nearest luxury hotel and march into theirs. If you walk in looking confident people rarely question you. The downside to changing outside the office is that you will have to carry your old work clothes with you all night.

Once in a bathroom, remove day make-up and immediately apply your moisturiser. Then wash under your arms (amazing how much fresher you will feel if you do this); if you can, also wash your feet. People may come in wondering what on earth you're on, but if you want to smell and look good for the man of your dreams do you really care if you end up with a reputation for being a bit quirky?

Once you're washed, brush your teeth, apply your make-up, then change your clothes, brush your hair, spray on some scent and you're ready. If you have about half an hour and your date is in a town or city, you might want to nip into a hairdresser's for a quick wash and blow dry. Then you can do your make-up there. But you should probably get the underarm and feet washing out of the way beforehand!

So that's the way you look dealt with. Now for your psyche; you need to shake away the office from your brain as well as your body. If you can find somewhere you're unlikely to be disturbed a good way to do this is to do some gentle stretching exercises. Stand up straight, reach your arms above your head and then breathe out as you reach for your toes. Breathe in once you're down there and clasp your ankles. Slowly breathe in as you bend you knees and breathe out as you straighten them, edging closer to the floor with each breath. Repeat this ten times and ignore any stressful thoughts that try to crowd your brain. Next raise your arms above your head, breathing out as you go up. Breathe in as you slowly lower your arms to your side. Repeat five times. Remember to focus on where you're going, who you're meeting and what you want out of the date...the office can wait until tomorrow.

'Be prepared.'
Motto of the Scout Association

Defining
idea...

15

How did it go?

Q How will I stay perky after a really busy day?

A   You'd be amazed what adrenalin does for you. A friend of mine recently had a hugely important date after a horrendous day that started with an overnight flight from New York, meetings all day and lunch with her boss. But the excitement of the date kept her going and by midnight she had so much adrenalin rushing around her system (along with some alcohol) that she was positively radiant. If you can't rely on natural adrenalin give your system a helping hand by downing some effervescent vitamin C tablets.

Q Anything else I can do to freshen up?

A   You could take some breath fresheners with you, and pop one in just a few minutes before you're due to meet. You can cut out the full change of clothes and just take another shirt or top with you. If you're a bloke you might want to think about at least bringing another pair of socks. Don't forget to dispose of the others somewhere though, you don't want her to come across them while seductively caressing you.

5

Cream's crackers

The number one beauty rule? Moisturise. Experts say keeping skin hydrated can help banish those dimples.

'Moisturise daily' is the kind of advice dispensed by both your mother and beauty experts at glossy magazines. And while you know it can be great for your face, will it really help reduce cellulite on your bum?

Skin specialists assure us it can. That's because when you slather on moisturiser, it helps plump out your skin. The effects may be temporary but adding moisture can smooth out those dimples and orange-peel bits to a degree.

The truth is cellulite looks worse on dehydrated or dry skin. That's because when your skin lacks moisture, it looks thinner, so those little pockets of fatty cells beneath the skin (which are the cellulite) are more noticeable. If you rehydrate your skin, you reduce the appearance of cellulite.

Most of us don't need to be reminded to moisturise our faces, but the skin on the rest of our body often gets neglected. So aim to moisturise day and night – after a shower in the morning or after your bedtime bath.

Here's an idea for you...

Add avocados to your shopping list. They're full of mono-unsaturated fats and vitamin E, which are good for your skin. They make a delicious snack or chuck a few slices in a sandwich or over a salad. You can even make a moisturising beauty mask with them. Simply mush up two or three avocados into a soft paste and smother over your bottom – massaging it in using circular movements with the avocado stone (or get a willing bystander to do this for you!) Then just wash it off with warm water.

Expensive, delicious smelling unguents make it a more pleasurable task, but any good moisturiser or body oil will do the trick.

Some of the best tried and tested brands of moisturisers include Dermalogica, Clarins, Decleor, and Nivea or Olay are great bargain buys. They make no claims about cellulite reduction, as they're simple body moisturisers, but with regular use, chances are your skin will look plumper and smoother and cellulite that bit less troublesome!

Moisturisers actually work by trapping the moisture into your skin (rather than adding moisture). But as you age, your skin thins and loses more moisture, so it's vital to use a good cream or lotion as the years go by. Even petroleum jelly (in Vaseline) works by trapping water into the skin, reducing water loss. And that doesn't cost an arm and a leg! That said, if splashing out on a pricey, beautifully packaged body moisturiser is going to make the entire process more pleasurable, then you may be more likely to build it into your regular toilette. And with moisturising, regularity is the key.

Other good tips to avoid dehydrating your skin is to avoid too hot water in your bath or shower as this can harm your body's lipids (natural fats). Don't soak for too long in hot water either. However sleepy or anxious you are to get between the sheets, make sure you do moisturise at night – experts say that's when the skin is more permeable so better able to absorb beneficial ingredients.

During dry weather or if you live in air-conditioned or centrally heated rooms, try using a humidifier to put moisture back into the air. Alternatively put a bowl of water on a radiator.

Defining idea...

Avoid over-using harsh soaps or detergent-based cleansers or bubble baths; these can strip the natural oils from your skin and make it drier. Experts say warm water is good enough to get your body clean – unless you're really grubby. Glycerine is a good ingredient to look for in soaps as this is really moisturising.

The sun is cruel to cellulite sufferers precisely because it conspires to dry out the skin, which makes those orange-peel dimples more noticeable.

When you lounge on your *chaise longue*, baking yourself in the sun, dangerous UV rays release nasty free radicals, which attack the collagen in your skin. This reduces its elasticity. On your face, this spells wrinkles. On your bottom and thighs it means skin becomes more saggy, less firm and plump. The reason that cellulite gets worse with age is because the collagen and elastin in your skin become weaker and less elastic – and when they're less pliable, the fatty pockets beneath the skin aren't held in place and become more noticeable.

Best advice, then, is to always use a sunscreen (make sure it's at least a factor 15) and use plenty of it. Reapply it often and stay out of the sun between noon and 3 p.m. – the hottest part of the day. And stick to fake tan, which is a great way to disguise cellulite.

How did
it go?

Q   **Is it true that it's more beneficial to apply moisturiser onto damp skin?**

A   *An old wives' tale, this one. The cream is actually diluted by the moisture on your skin, so you're effectively reducing the richness of the cream or lotion. Instead wait until you're properly dry before you slather it on.*

Q   **What about exfoliators? Do they do any good?**

A   *Again, there are temporary benefits. Exfoliating is a great way to brighten up the skin as it removes the dead surface skin cells, which can make skin look dull and lacklustre. When these surface skin cells are removed, the skin looks smoother instantly. When your skin is smooth, fake tan goes on more evenly – and we all know cellulite is less noticeable when your body's beautifully bronzed.*

6

Quick fixes

Puffy eyes? Dark circles? Frizzy hair? Try these instant beautifiers for those hot date emergencies.

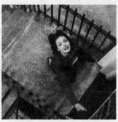

You know how it is. A huge bouquet of plump pink roses lands on your desk at work with a note saying, 'Darling, meet me at Claridges at eight. Wear something irresistible.'

In my dreams! Nevertheless, there *are* moments when we need to look super-gorgeous fast, like for a last-minute party, date or business lunch, for example. And since they'll undoubtedly arise on a bad nail, spot or hair day, here are some troubleshooting tips to catch the beauty demons off guard.

COVER UP THOSE SPOTS

First, clean the spot area using cotton wool and a medicated lotion. Next, apply a mattifying product or gel to the area to remove any excess oil and prevent your concealer from sliding off. Pick a concealer that's the same colour as your face, ideally dry in texture rather than creamy, and apply it right in the middle of the spot. Using a brush or your middle finger, wipe away any excess. Remember, you're trying to camouflage the spot, not the area around it.

Here's an idea for you... **For posh nails cut corners with press-on falsies. Pick the pre-glued ones and simply press them on over your natural nails. They should last up to three days.**

INSTANTLY BOOST YOUR COMPLEXION

Exfoliating to remove the layer of dead skin cells that dulls your complexion is the easiest way to brighten your skin and make you feel perkier. Splashing your face with cold water is a great pick-me-up, too. Beauty doyenne Eve Lom (www.evelom.co.uk) has her own method. Start by massaging in a rich oil-based cleanser and then remove it using a muslin cloth. Next, massage cleanser over your face and neck gently, applying deep pressure with the pads of your fingertips. Start behind the ears to stimulate the lymphatic system, relieve congestion and reduce fluid. Repeat this three times, then rinse the cloth, rub off the cleanser and splash your face with cold water.

FIX PUFFY EYES

Give yourself a mini lymphatic drainage massage to help beat the fluid retention. Tap your middle finger around each eye in circular movements, then lie down and place cotton wool pads soaked in witch hazel or rosewater over your eyes. Alternatively, try damp camomile teabags that have been cooled in the fridge. Drink plenty of water too as dehydration can make puffy eyes worse. If you've time a quick workout can help boost circulation and lymph drainage. As a long-term solution, sleep with your head raised higher than your body.

BRIGHTEN DARK CIRCLES

These nasties occur when your blood vessels become visible through your skin. Some people have naturally thin skin, but you do lose fat in this area as you age, so they tend to get worse. Start in the corner of your eye and apply concealer a shade lighter than your skin tone. Ideally, choose cream concealer as it's easier to apply and goes on more evenly. Some experts say that eye creams containing vitamin K, which helps boost blood flow, can help with dark circles.

'Illusions are the mirages of Hope.'
ANONYMOUS

Defining idea...

TAME FRIZZINESS

You may have been born with frizzy hair. Or too much sun, too many colourants, blow-drying at too high a temperature and the need for a jolly good trim have left it crispy or wayward. Aim to condition your hair regularly and book that haircut if it's overdue. If you're on the point of going out use a leave-in conditioner before you blow-dry or add a few drops of smoothing serum that contains panthenol or silicone-based products to coat the cuticle and help it lie flat. Don't be afraid to spritz your hair with hairspray either as it will help prevent moisture in humid air (which causes your hair to frizz) from penetrating your hair.

GLAM UP YOUR HAIR

'Women have two weapons – cosmetics and tears.'
ANONYMOUS

Defining idea...

Try this super speedy blow-dry. Lightly spray your hair with water then add a root-lifting product to give you instant body and volume.
Start by blow-drying your roots, lifting the hair upwards as you go. Then smooth your hair into style using a natural bristle brush to give you extra shine. Finally, use your fingers to tousle your hair into a dishevelled but glam style, spray some perfume in the air and 'walk' into it. Instant gorgeousness.

How did it go?

Q   **Unfortunately, I don't have visible cheekbones. Short of lipo, surgery or starvation, what can I do to 'fake' them?**

A   *Using a concealer that's a shade lighter than your skin, carefully blend from the edge of your eye upwards. Since light reflects higher on your face, this will create the illusion of higher cheekbones.*

Q   **Any quickies for enhancing my eyes?**

A   *Yes. Here's a sixty-second job that will accentuate eyes of any colour. Dabbing your regular lipgloss along your upper lashes using a clean fingertip or cotton bud will make your eyes sheer and shimmery and give them a natural twinkle.*

Q   **I often smudge or dent my nails right after I've painted them. Is there any way I can salvage them without having to start from scratch?**

A   *To help even out the surface use your finger to apply a tiny drop of polish remover to your nail and lightly smooth it over the dent, smudge or crease. Once it's dry, seal it with a thin layer of topcoat.*

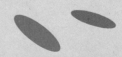

7

The tan commandments

Having a tan makes you look thinner, healthier and sexier. There really is no downside – lookswise. But healthwise, you have to prepare yourself for the beach.

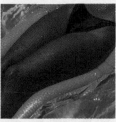

So we've all heard about the dental floss look on Copacabana Beach. That minuscule, almost invisible bikini all those hot Brazilian chicks wear.

But how would you look in one of those while sunning yourself in Norfolk? (An unlikely thought in itself.) It's no good just exposing that wobbly white flesh and hoping you'll leave the beach looking like Halle Berry. You'll look more like a boiled lobster. You need to prepare yourself for the suntan and this can take weeks of forward planning.

You need to prepare your skin, especially if it's fair. Some people take beta carotene pills for a few weeks before they go on holiday. This substance can help you go brown and can be found in carrots and other brightly coloured vegetables as well as the pills. You should exfoliate before you expose your skin to the sun. This removes dead skin and makes the tan more even. Try body brushing or use exfoliating creams. Once on holiday be sure to put on sunscreen before tanning and not just

Here's an idea for you...

Try bleaching the body hair that you're holding on to before you start sunbathing. That way they will be lovely and blonde, making you look even more tanned and gorgeous, and you won't be self conscious about them. Jolen Cream Bleach is the best one.

when you've burnt (when it's too late). Sunscreens should be applied about half an hour before you go outside. During the first few days, limit your tanning sessions to 20 minutes and avoid the sun between 11.30 and 2.30. You must moisturise all the time, use a good aftersun product in the evening and keep piling on that cream during the day. The sun drinks the moisture from your skin. It also removes collagen, the substance that gives your skin elasticity. So you need to make sure you take plenty of vitamin C while on holiday as your body can't produce collagen without it.

Tanned skin is damaged skin and the more you expose the skin to the sun the more damaged it will become over time. No wonder so many people swear by fake tan. Products are improving all the time so if you purchase and apply wisely you should be able to avoid the dreaded streaks. To ensure even colour remember to exfoliate before applying the fake tan and apply sparingly to areas like knees and elbows. Either wear special fake tanning gloves or wash the palms of your hands thoroughly after applying.

You also need to prepare your body. This means a diet and a strict exercise regime at least two months before you plan to wear that dental floss. In terms of what to wear on the beach, this obviously depends on who you're holidaying with and where you're going. In Rio one can definitely get away with a minuscule bikini. They wear practically nothing there, even the women without great bodies. Somehow they get away with it, they move well, are tanned and confident.

The only thing to avoid is looking cheap. You can always wear the minuscule bikini while lying around trying to catch the rays but cover up with a sarong when you're wandering about. A classic swimming costume can be extremely elegant and sexy too, don't assume that in the beachwear stakes less is always more.

Don't forget your hair. Sea water and sun can take their toll. Give it a deep conditioning treatment every time you wash it. Comb the conditioner through carefully and wrap your hair in a hot towel. If you're trying to go blonde then squeeze lemon juice into it for some natural and cheap highlights. But don't forget to condition it well every day as lemon juice has a drying effect.

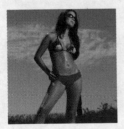

'Summertime and the livin' is easy.'
HEYWARD and GERSHWIN,
American songwriters.

Defining idea...

27

How did
it go?

Q   **Can't I just cover myself in oil for that really sexy look?**

A   *Of course. Once the sun has gone down. But during the day you need a proper sun cream. Oil will attract the sun and you'll literally fry. If you live in a warm climate (or even during the summer months in the UK) you should wear a moisturiser with an SPF of at least 15 to protect your face. It is recommended that you throw away old sunscreens and buy new ones every year since the effect of the heat will make them basically useless the following season. A bit expensive, but there are so many new improved products out you might want a change anyway.*

Q   **If I wear suntan lotion every time I'm never going to get brown in two weeks. How can I look gorgeous?**

A   *But you might look better at fifty. Sun-damaged skin looks rough, red and puffy. And that's just before we start on the risk of skin cancer. No one wants to be a killjoy but there's evidence that binge-tanning – really going for it for just a few weeks a year – carries more risk of cancer than exposure over a longer period.*

8

Get the most out of your holiday

There's nothing like a fortnight in the sun to make you feel more gorgeous, so why not book one today? It's therapy.

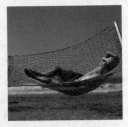

The key to a successful holiday is to extract the maximum benefit you possibly can from them, while paying very little yourself. Here's how.

EAT LIKE A MEDITERRANEAN

We all know that holidays can be great for our looks. There's usually a choice of delicious new foods to be sampled, so while you're away make a conscious effort to eat better – lots of wholegrains, fruit, vegetables and proteins such as lean meat and fish. That way you'll be getting a wider range of vitamins and minerals.

Make dining a special experience. Take pleasure in setting the table and preparing the food. If you really relish what you're eating you'll eat less, as it takes twenty minutes for the brain to learn that you're full. And no reading or watching TV or

Here's an idea for you...

Eat like you're on a Caribbean holiday and spice up your home cooking by adding the herbs and spices used in exotic food. Spices also make a healthy alternative to salt. Cinnamon, allspice and cloves provide antioxidants, ginger aids digestion and garlic boosts heart health.

standing up while you're eating, or munching on the run. The idea is to savour the smells, sensations and colours of the food, and to slow down to help digestion.

Also, aim to drink more water. This shouldn't be hard as you'll want to stay cool poolside, but make sure you at least match every alcoholic drink with a glass of water. Try, too, to make time for breakfast. This shouldn't be difficult either as it is such a treat to linger over breakfast, rather than having to run out to work with a piece of toast in your handbag. Plus nutritionists say that breakfast is one of the best ways to control your weight and boost your metabolism.

EXPLORE, CREATE, DREAM

There's nothing like a holiday somewhere exotic and/or romantic for firing up your passions. The sun, food, architecture, history or the region can all stir up your imagination and rekindle your *joie de vivre*. Capitalise on this and don't merely bury yourself in your Jilly Cooper novel.

Use your holiday as a springboard for new beginnings. If you're thinking of making a career change or redecorating the spare room, now's the time to do the groundwork. While you're on your chaise longue, make a couple of to-do lists; things to do today, this month, this year, that you want to achieve before you're thirty/forty/married/infirm, whatever. It could be a safari in Africa, losing 5 kg or running a marathon. This is an extremely motivating exercise, plus you'll feel great as you tick things off your list. Think back to ambitions you had as a young 'un. Have they changed or have you neglected them? It's never too late to learn something new, see another continent, write your first novel, etc. The more fulfilled you are in life, the more confident and contented you'll appear – and 100% more attractive to boot!

MOVE THAT BEACH BODY

We tend to spend most of our holiday outdoors, soaking up rays. However, rather than surgically attaching yourself to a deckchair, aim to incorporate at least thirty minutes of strenuous activity into your day. Swim, try windsurfing or diving, run on the beach, play Frisbee – anything that gets your heart rate pumping. And use your holiday to strengthen your relationship. Use the extra time you have for talking, sightseeing, taking up new hobbies together or inspecting the hotel linen together. Get motivated!

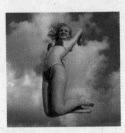

'Come, woo me, woo me; for now I am in a holiday humour, and like enough to consent.'
SHAKESPEARE

Defining
idea...

31

How did it go?

Q **How can I avoid insect bites? I'm always eaten alive wherever I go, whether it's Bermuda or Bognor!**

A *Interestingly, gnats, mozzies and midges are attracted to bright clothing and tend to go out to eat at dusk, which coincides nicely with Happy Hour. The best natural pesticides are citronella candles or citronella essential oil. Alternatively, try a mosquito coil or slather yourself in insect repellent. If you're bitten, you should find that an antihistamine will soothe the area.*

Q **What is it with flip-flops? They always give me blisters.**

A *The skin between your big toe and second toe is very sensitive, so it's little wonder that all that chafing irritates your skin and causes blisters. Try rubbing Vaseline between your toes to help prevent those sore patches.*

Q **How can I prevent post-holiday blues?**

A *Plan another one soon. Also, schedule regular 'me time' for the weeks ahead that might include evening classes, gym sessions or relaxing nights in with a video and a glass of wine. Fill up your diary with good things like music, food and fun people, and declutter your surroundings or tart up your bedroom or living room. Book a fake tan treatment for a couple of weeks after your return as your real one will be fading and this will help you retain that holiday high.*

9

Dress for success

Clothing communicates, it's a simple fact. No matter how much we regard ourselves as able to look behind the façade, one of the first signifiers we read is the packaging.

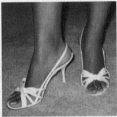

And getting yours right is key when trying to attract the right kind of attention. So exactly what is the right kind of attention?

Basically, you need to dress for the kind of man you want to appeal to, and for the kind of relationship you want to establish. Looking for a playful fling? As long as you aren't wearing a bin bag, it almost doesn't matter what you have on as you know what you want. Looking for a fellow art buff for a meaningful, life-long relationship? A spandex off-the-shoulder, thigh-skimming tube dress with some plastic wet-look boots may make other viewers at the private view think you are a performance artist. Or whatever. But you might at least earn your bus fare home.

WHAT HAPPENED TO SELF-RESPECT?

Dressing to attract a man might sound like the past hundred years of women's liberation never happened. But the fact is, wearing your favourite neck-to-ankle baggy jumper may make you feel secure but it does not, in any way whatsoever, say

Think about how your outfits are received; you may think you are being the belle of the ball but actually be coming on like a train. Consider the type of event you are going to and not just the impression you would like to make. A Halloween house party might be more suited to a fun homemade tramp outfit than an expensively hired catsuit; nothing says 'Look at me, I'm desperate!' like a bid to be super-sexy at all times. One quiet Saturday afternoon, try on lots of clothes and find something that is flattering, a little sexy and comfortable; then hang it on the back of the bedroom door as your SOS date outfit, if you get panicked. If in doubt, default to a little black dress. These have served womankind well for a very long time.

that you are available or interested in taking things to a romantic level. Sexual attraction is an important part of finding a partner and there is nothing wrong with it: so get with the programme, have a good think about your best bits and pieces, and get them out.

FEELING FINE

So how do you get the balance between what you feel comfortable in and what you think might attract the right man? Firstly, you must feel comfortable in whatever you wear, as that will help radiate confidence and an ease with your body. And don't try anything frighteningly new or too high fashion; lots of men don't care that your shoes are the latest catwalk chic, but they might care if you take a head-first dive down the club steps because you haven't mastered the art of walking in them.

A LITTLE BIT OF WHAT YOU FANCY...

It never hurts to advertise, and men are basically visual creatures, so a glimpse of a taut thigh, a crisp white shirt with a flattering neckline or a well-turned ankle in some killer heels are all great tools in your armoury.

'Put even the plainest woman into a beautiful dress and unconsciously she will try to live up to it.'
LADY DUFF GORDON, 20s fashion designer

Defining idea...

However, there is a fine line between being tantalising and being tarty. This is where the 'one or the other' rule comes into play. If you have a great décolletage, feel free to hoist your boobs up and dab some seductive scent in pertinent places. However, you may want to team that stunning, sparkly, low-cut top with some simple flattering black trousers, rather than a denim skirt the size of a belt. Even if you also have fabulous legs, too much of a good thing can slide into slut. So choose one good area and work it to its best advantage.

Now consider where you are going. A miniskirt with a black polo neck is a winning combination if you have devastating legs, but not if you have to hide all your assets under the table during dinner, with you now looking like a severe intellectual beatnik about to grill him on existentialism. The same miniskirt worn in the gods at the theatre might get the audience looking in the opposite direction from the stage. Be as objective as you can; you might love that skirt to bits, but if it's not going to work for you, put it back in the wardrobe.

How did it go?

Q **I've got a first date with a guy that I met through work but I've very little to go on; I haven't even seen him out of a suit. What shall I wear?**

A *Ah, so you know he's interested, because you are on this date in the first place. But now you have the real stress of coming up with a winning fashion combination. In an information void, the best thing to do is pick your favourite outfit, one that you feel attractive in, and play it by ear.*

Q **But what if he's a rugger-bugger sweatshirt wearer, and hates my retro 70s cowgirl thing?**

A *If there's enough going on to think you can get through dinner together, then there should be enough to get you on to the next date. If you hate his outfit but think he's great you have two options – you can stop being so shallow, or you can get familiar with the boil-wash cycle on the washing machine. It was designed for weeding out bad jumpers in a non-confrontational manner.*

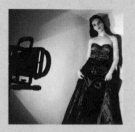

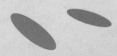

10

Beauty sleep

There's nothing more delicious and restorative than a good night's sleep. Here's how to track one down tonight.

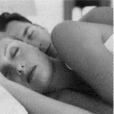

You only need a few late nights combined with early mornings to realise just why they call it 'beauty sleep'. Lack of shuteye usually means waking up with grey, pasty skin, lacklustre lips and a short fuse.

That's because vital repair work goes on when we're asleep and as we pass through its different stages, our skin gets replenished and our body's growth hormone is produced to help repair and regenerate all our cells. Sleep also enables us to process the information we've accumulated in the day; without it our brain simply doesn't function effectively. In addition, a lack of sleep will affect our immune system, making us more susceptible to infections. It can also cause us to put on weight since when we're tired our willpower is weakened and we're more likely to skip exercise and reach for fatty, sugary or salty foods.

Here's an idea for you...

Instead of one hour's kip take a far more refreshing fifteen-minute power nap, ideally between 2 p.m. and 4 p.m. when your body is primed for sleep. If you're at work give yourself time out for ten minutes and put your head on your desk, close your eyes and focus on slowing your breathing and emptying your mind.

HOW MUCH SLEEP DO WE REALLY NEED?

Some people thrive on very few hours, but most of us need between six and eight hours to feel refreshed. Most experts say that seven is the optimum amount.

WHAT IF SLUMBER IS EVADING YOU?

Here are ten ways to ensure a better night's sleep.

1. Stick to a routine

The best way to guarantee restful sleep is to stick to a regular time for both going to bed and waking up. Don't make the mistake of thinking you can catch up on your sleep at weekends by having a lie-in till midday, as this will only disrupt your pattern and may explain why so many of us find it harder to get to sleep on Sunday nights. Go to bed and get up at the same time every day, including weekends, and if you must lie in, just allow yourself an extra hour.

2. Try earplugs

If your partner or the neighbours are conspiring against you, just block them out. If you're woken in the middle of a sleep cycle (a sleep cycle lasts about an hour and a half) by outside noise, you'll feel very sluggish and feel like you have a hangover – which is particularly grim on top of a real hangover.

3. Try lavender

Lavender is a well-known traditional remedy for insomnia and it has actually been scientifically proven to have a sedative effect on your brain. Try sprinkling some on a hanky, pillow or pyjamas.

4. Eat for a good night's sleep

Avoid rich food at night and wait two hours after a heavy meal before going to bed. Try a carbohydrate-rich snack before bedtime, such as some crackers or a piece of toast, as carbohydrates release serotonin, which can help you feel relaxed.

5. Keep your bedroom for sleeping (or sex)

Never work, eat or watch television in bed.

6. Sleep in the right position

According to Chinese wisdom, the best position for restful sleep is on your right side, in a foetal position, with your legs slightly apart and your right arm resting in front of the pillow. This position is said to allow your blood to circulate freely.

'Eating fish with green vegetables for dinner will promote a good night's sleep as these foods are rich in calcium and magnesium, necessary both for brain chemistry balance and to relax the body.'
IAN MARBER, food doctor

Defining idea...

39

7. Keep your bed spartan

Rather than tons of pillows, stick to crisp sheets and cool, loose pyjamas. Keep a window open if it's warm as a lower body temperature promotes sleep.

8. Keep out of the wind

If you're prone to bloating, avoid cruciferous vegetables such as cauliflower, cabbage and broccoli in the evening as they can make you too windy to sleep.

9. Relax

Keep a notepad by the bed for jotting down all those worries or additions to your to-do list which often invade your head when you're trying to drop off. Write them down and then let them go.

10. Relax

Take slow, deep breaths through your nostrils and out through your mouth and focus on your diaphragm as it moves up and down. Try breathing in for about four seconds and then out for another four seconds. Let go of each limb, each muscle, until your entire body is relaxed. Mentally scan your body for tense bits and exaggerate each area until it's tight and uncomfortable then release.

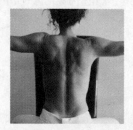
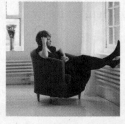

Q   Do you know of any good drug-free sedatives?

A   Try some of the many over-the-counter herbal remedies. Valerian has long been used as a sedative and it can have positive effects on mild insomnia. It also has very few side effects. Alternatively, investigate acupuncture, which can also help you get to sleep more easily.

Q   Can you really sleep too much?

A   Yes! Your sleep consists of ninety-minute cycles of both light and deep sleep. Your body tends to wake up at the end of one of these ninety-minute cycles, so if you extend your sleeping hours and wake up mid-cycle, you can end up feeling groggier and puffy-eyed. Try to stick to a routine.

Q   Is a nightcap a good idea?

A   Sorry, no. Alcohol may make you feel sleepy at first, but it's actually a stimulant so your slumber will be disturbed. Instead, stick to camomile tea or warm milk with a teaspoon of honey (honey is a natural sedative).

How did
it go?

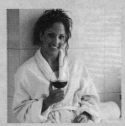

41

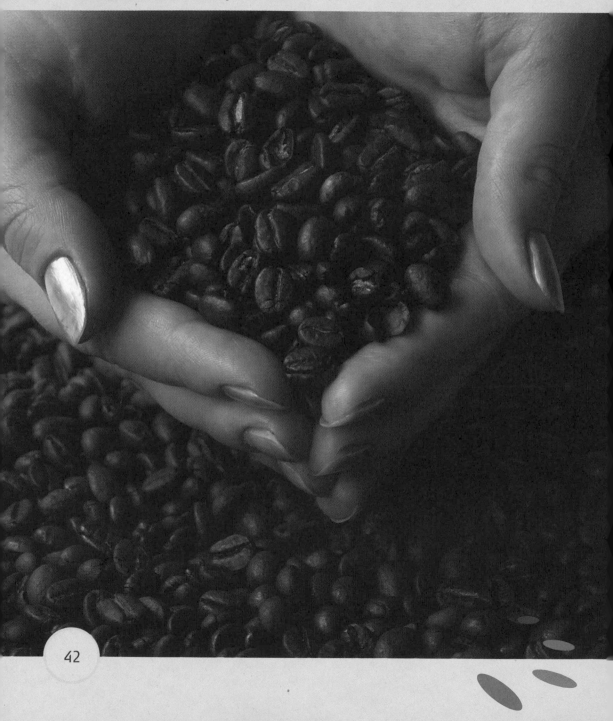

11

Beans means lines

Caffeine can dehydrate and age the skin, which can make cellulite worse. If you're a coffee fiend, it's time to switch to decaf.

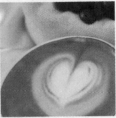

This will hurt if you're one of those people who can't face life without an espresso or five. But that black stuff is no friend to your behind.

OK, most of us tend to find that a little caffeine fix makes us feel more alert, better able to concentrate and less tired. But too much caffeine can lead to anxiousness, restlessness, leave you feeling jittery and unable to sleep – and give you headaches, nausea or palpitations.

But you want to know what caffeine has to do with cellulite, and more importantly why your behind might thank you for cutting back on the cappuccino.

Firstly, caffeine can contribute to weight gain. (And there we were, thinking our little black cup was helping get us into our little black dress! *Au contraire*.) Apparently drinking two cups of coffee is enough to raise the levels of the stress hormone cortisol and insulin in your body, which is thought to accelerate ageing and encourage the body to store fat. Studies have shown that when coffee drinkers

Here's an idea for you...

Ditch that coffee and instead try starting your day with a large glass of freshly squeezed orange juice and a bowl of berries. This will boost your intake of vitamin C, which is important for the production of collagen and can strengthen the capillaries, which feed the skin. And better skin means smoother thighs.

reduce their coffee intake, they lose weight, although it's not yet understood why this happens.

Plus when our blood sugar levels are raised and our insulin levels are disrupted, we're more likely to be tempted by sugary treats – that espresso may lead to a choccy croissant or two.

Caffeine is also bad for your skin because it impedes your blood circulation. Skin requires a regular blood supply to stay looking young and healthy. A lack of oxygen can lead to dark circles, puffiness, fine lines, poor colour. You know how your face looks after too many espressos and a few late nights...well, the skin on your behind is also being robbed of vital nutrients too, which means it's going to look dry and dehydrated – and that will make your cellulite worse.

Caffeine also contributes to water retention; as it's a diuretic, it can dehydrate your body. When you're dehydrated, cells hold on to water – and your fat cells hold on to fluids, which, on your bottom and thighs, make your skin bulge out and look puffier and more dimply.

And if that hasn't put you off the black stuff, bear in mind it's also no friend if you're a PMS sufferer. That's because caffeine increases sleeplessness, anxiety and tension, which are symptoms of PMS. A study of over 200 college-age women found severe PMS symptoms in 60% of those who drank more than four cups of caffeinated drinks a day. Coffee also causes your body to get rid of important nutrients, especially B vitamins, which are needed for energy, good skin and hair, healthy growth, and mood.

It gets worse. Caffeine also destroys calcium – one cup of coffee removes about 6 mg of calcium from your body's stores. Experts have found that calcium is important in weight loss because it's thought to help prevent fat storage and boost metabolism. (You can increase your calcium in your diet with skimmed milk, cheddar cheese, fish, sesame seeds and dried figs. Other good sources include steamed tofu and nuts.)

'Behind every successful woman is a substantial amount of coffee.'
STEPHANIE PIRO, artist

Defining idea...

So how much is too much? How much caffeine are *you* drinking?

About 300 mg caffeine a day is 'a moderate' intake. One 190 ml cup of instant coffee contains about 100 mg, tea has 30–60 mg per cup and cola around 50 mg per can. So three mugs of tea per day plus one cup of coffee would give you almost your daily 'allowance'.

Best advice, then, is to cut down as much as you can – don't drink more than one or two cups a day – and look instead for healthy alternatives.

Bear in mind that chocolate also contains caffeine; in fact there's about 10 mg of caffeine in 50 g of milk chocolate – dark chocolate contains 28 mg per 50 g. There's more caffeine in a 125 g (4 oz) bar of dark chocolate than in a cup of instant coffee...so if you're serious about getting rid of cellulite, go easy on the chocolate.

How did
it go?

Q   **OK, you've convinced me. So are there any good alternatives to coffee?**

A   *Try dandelion tea. Dandelion is rich in potassium and has been used as a purifying tonic. You can buy ready-made teabags, or, alternatively, brew your own: pour boiling water over two teaspoons of dried dandelion leaves (or four teaspoons of freshly chopped) and steep for ten minutes. Strain, and drink. Or try green tea. It's made from the unfermented leaves of the tea plant, and has half the caffeine of coffee. It's rich in antioxidants, which can help mop up the free radicals that are associated with ageing. If you can only replace one cup of coffee with a cup of green tea you'll be doing your body a favour. Redbush tea is another good alternative. It contains on average less than half the tannin of regular tea. Research shows it's rich in disease-fighting antioxidants quercetin and luteolin. Plus it helps your body absorb vitamin C better. And it's delicious.*

Q   **Help, I just can't give up my morning cup of coffee. How can I wake myself up without it?**

A   *If you can't switch to decaf, or really can't function rationally without a morning brew, try to increase your intake of fluids. So for every caffeine-containing drink (such as tea, coffee or cola), make sure you have at least half a cup of water to counteract the diuretic effect.*

46

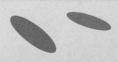

12

The shock of the old

Growing older is part of life. Smoking gets you there quicker than if you don't.

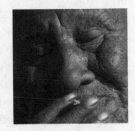

Not wanting to quit to protect your lungs or heart? Seeing the impact smoking has on your face and body should give you the needed push.

Smoking kills. Every smoker knows that smoking kills. Indeed, dicing with death, when the real prospect of dying seems a lifetime away, is part of the initial thrill of smoking. It gives the habit its edge and glamour, and makes those who smoke feel that little bit more alive and interesting than the sensible types who don't.

Smoking also ages its consumers. A recent research paper in *The Lancet*, one of the world's foremost medical journals, found that someone smoking a packet of twenty cigarettes a day for forty years had at sixty the body of a non-smoker aged sixty-seven and a half. Scientific evidence that deep down even the most hardened and unapologetic smoker knows to be true. The evidence of the ageing effect of smoking is everywhere, even staring out of the chap you shave in the morning or the woman to whose face you apply lipstick.

Here's an idea for you...

Talk to a selection of children and teenagers who don't know anything about you (if you dare). Ask them to tell you how old you are – the first number that occurs to them, not a figure to flatter you. You may be shocked to discover that this group think you're older than you are. Adults are more likely to tell you what they think you want to hear.

The question then becomes how you can convert insights like these into motivation providing the impetus to help you quit. The good news is that by quitting now you can move out of the ageing fast lane already congested with other smokers and back in the middle lane, and start rubbing shoulders with those smug, healthy sons of bitches who know how to say no.

COMPARE AND CONTRAST

You might have seen those magazine articles that look at the effect a healthy lifestyle has on individuals. Often what is most striking is the illustrations which compare fit and unfit couples. By early middle age there is already a striking difference. The fit couple weigh less, and have better posture, skin, muscle tone and stamina. They look younger than the artist's impression of the other couple. If you think this is pushing the bounds of reality, take a look at a non-smoking sibling and ask yourself seriously whether they are wearing better than you are.

DOCTORING PHOTOGRAPHS

You're an only child or all your siblings smoke. No worries: doctor, a photo please. Take a recent snap of your head and shoulders, enlarge it and then trace over. On your traced sketch add additional wrinkles around the eyes, forehead, mouth and so on. Add or extend a double chin, thin out the hair. What should emerge is an image of yourself in years to come. While there is no way yet of reversing this process, its speed can be checked by quitting cigarettes.

You are likely to get an even more painful image of your future using a computer software tool like Photoshop. It's widely available, so if you don't have the program, there are sure to be plenty of people who'd be willing to take this project on for you. With a little imagination they can yellow your teeth, make your skin more flawed, and lighten and thin your hair. The more advanced users will have no difficulty extending and deepening crows feet eyes, your frown and other tell-tell signs of ageing. In fact, this process is just reversing the doctoring taking place in magazines all the time. Print out and display in a prominent position.

> *'One only dies once, and it's for such a long time.'*
> MOLIÈRE

Defining idea...

PAVEMENT PORTRAIT PAINTERS

> *'My face looks like a wedding cake left out in the rain.'*
> W.H. AUDEN

Defining idea...

In most large cities, shopping malls and tourists traps you can find an artist sitting behind an easel surrounded by images of James Dean, Madonna, John Wayne, Jack Nicholson, and current sporting and pop icons. Whether these drawings were actually undertaken by the artist in front of you is not a subject for this book. Most, however, can draw a flattering portrait of their sitter. Indeed, their artistic skills are usually exceeded by an ability to delude the sitter into accepting a flattering likeness.

Your purpose is to commission a portrait that adds a decade or two to how you look now. If the artist does not appear to understand, say that you want to see what you will look like in ten or twenty years' time.

Take your picture home and frame it, having written in large capitals the words: STOPPING SMOKING WILL SLOW DOWN THE TIME IT TAKES TO GET TO THIS. You could also photocopy it to hang in every room of your house.

How did it go?

Q **When I want to look younger all I have to do is put on the old war paint. I'm pushing forty and can still turn heads, so this idea seems pretty pointless for me. Tell me why I should stop?**

A *Time marches on. All we're suggesting is that stopping smoking slows down the ravages of time. Make-up can cover up a lot of blemishes, but you're on a diminishing return. And there'll come the day when you'll have to start using a trowel to put it on.*

Q **I did what you suggested and gave a mate of mine a digital photo which he worked on for a few hours. In the picture I look just like my mother's eldest brother. It gave me quite a shock, as he died when I was only eight. My kids thought it was really funny and suggested I get a haircut like him and start wearing his sort of clothes. Apart from providing harmless entertainment for my kids, how does this idea help?**

A *You are what you eat; likewise, your body bears witness to everything you do to it. Without getting too high-handed, non-smokers generally wear better than smokers, and my suggestions here are a way of reminding you that you are no different from anyone else. Being reminded about someone in the family whose life was shortened by smoking is a bit of a wake-up call.*

13

Luscious lips

Want plump, bee-stung, kissable lips? Before facing the needle try a few simple tips on how to fake them.

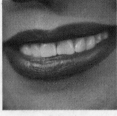

We can't all do pillar-box lips. Bold colours emphasise less than perfect lips but if you haven't the colouring or the requisite attitude, red lipstick can look more hooker than siren. Still, there's plenty you can do to enhance your pout.

SIZE UP YOUR LIPS

Assess their shape. You can minimise a large mouth and lips that are too full by choosing a neutral tone of lipstick. Use a lipliner to draw a line just inside the lips and choose a dark shade of lipstick to fill, which will help to make them look smaller. Stay clear of dark colours if your lips are thin, as they'll make them look even smaller. Instead, use a lipliner to draw a line just over your natural lip line to create the illusion of fuller lips and then go for a bright colour to plump them up even more. Glossy or pearl lipsticks can also make lips look fuller, as they reflect the light.

Here's an idea for you...

To get whiter-looking teeth go for berries, plums and blue-based red lipsticks. The contrast will help make your teeth appear whiter and brighter. Avoid any yellow- or orange-based shades, including corals and browny colours, as they can make your teeth look yellow.

SELECT THE RIGHT SHADE OF LIPPY

Experts say that olive skins look their best next to berry shades. If your complexion and hair are fair, stick to reds with pinkish undertones. If you have pale skin and dark hair you'll find that strong, bright-red lipstick can look amazing. And if your skin is dark, then pick deep, rich reds.

PAY YOUR LIPS DUE SERVICE

Take the time to care for your lips in the same way that you care for your skin. Gently buff them with a soft, baby's toothbrush to remove dry skin and boost the circulation, then regularly apply lip balm. This is also a great way to soften up dry, cracked lips.

Defining idea...

'Beauty, to me, is about being comfortable in your own skin. That, or a kick-ass red lipstick.'
GWYNETH PALTROW

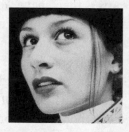

TRY THE BEE-STUNG LOOK

There's an art to perfecting bee-stung lips, so even those of us with thin lips can pout with the best of them. Try this:

1. First, outline your lips using a lip pencil in the same shade as your lipstick or lighter (never darker, unless you're a lap dancer or would like to be mistaken for one).
2. Then, using a lip brush, 'fill in' your lips. Instead of using a block of matt colour, build up gradually using a sheer lipstick. That way you'll capture the light, which will make your lips look fuller and plumper. Using a highlighter pen, draw a fine line around your upper lip, just above your Cupid's bow. Alternatively, try blending little dots of reflective foundation on your upper lip, which will also help accentuate a natural pout.
3. Finish with a dab of lipgloss on the fullest part of your lips.

Q   How do I make my lipstick last longer?

How did it go?

A   *You can find plenty of long-lasting formulations at the beauty counter these days. They can be drying, though, so prime your lips beforehand. First, dab some petroleum jelly on your lips and blot with a tissue. Then outline your lips with a lip pencil, apply the lipstick, blot with a tissue then add another coat. The lipstick should last for hours because it's effectively stained the lips. Plus, if you use a lipliner before applying your lipstick, you'll get a longer-lasting and even colour because you'll 'fill in' all those minute nooks and crannies.*

Q   Do I really need an SPF lip balm in the summer? Won't Vaseline stop them drying out?

A   *Vaseline won't stop lips from getting sunburnt. As your lips don't contain much melanin and the skin is thinnest here, they're more vulnerable to sun damage, so be sure to wear a protective balm with an SPF 15 in the summer, when you're skiing or in extremes of temperature. Lipsticks offer some protection, especially darker colours, but make sure you apply it regularly.*

Q   Is there a colour that suits everyone?

A   *Some experts say that plum lipstick suits everyone. It's particularly flattering on those with blue eyes as it really enhances the blue.*

Q   What's the best way to remove lipstick?

A   *A regular cleanser ought to do it. If you've been wearing a very dark colour that has stained your lips, eye make-up remover on a cotton pad should do the trick.*

14

The confidence factor

The trick to being sexy is to be confident. You need to believe in and accept yourself. There are of course bits of you that you don't like, but don't dwell on them. Exaggerate your good points and work on the bad ones.

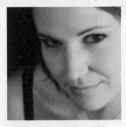

When you walk into a room imagine you are Jennifer Lopez or Tom Cruise; don't think 'God I look like a drowned rat and no one will find me attractive'.

Sex appeal is not just skin deep, it's also a question of attitude. Confidence is fundamental to sexiness and some people ooze it. They are magnetic, captivating and not necessarily drop-dead gorgeous. These are usually people that are open, gregarious, amusing and positive. All attributes which require confidence.

There are days when you will feel like you rule the world and days when you wonder why on earth anyone ever speaks to you. When you have days like the latter, try to think of them as bad hair days. Everyone has them, but they don't last for ever. Think to yourself: there are lots of good things about me. You could even make a list of all your achievements such as owning your home, holding down a

Here's an idea for you...

Write down the five things that most attract you to someone. And then work out how you can adapt them to work for you. For example, someone might have a very sexy tone of voice that you could imitate or maybe a way of sitting that is attractive. Practise small things like this and you'll already feel sexier and more confident.

job, an address book full of friends, a contented cat. Don't forget your best physical attributes. Noting them yourself almost by magic appears to flag them up to other people. Soon you'll be receiving compliments.

Set yourself small, achievable goals every week, and use them to boost your self-esteem and confidence (it's not just Americans who can get away with this). Or you could read self-help books. You've made a start by reading this idea so think of some other area of your life you can improve to make you sexier and then get thee to a bookshop (or try out some more Brilliant Ideas).

Try to look at yourself like a stock. Your share price will go up or down, depending on market perception. If things are going well, and you're on a high, your stock will soar; everyone wants to know you. If you're at a low then your price will drop. And you won't help this drop in price by moping around refusing to go out. You need to work at it until your share price is right up there again. A new haircut, a new outfit, a new career move, anything that will boost you over the bad period. So here are my top five tips for becoming more confident or feigning confidence:

1. Think about your good points and accentuate them. If you have lovely eyes, say, use them when you're talking to people or flirting.

2. Similarly, DO NOT think about your bad points. You may think the spot just under your chin is the most dramatically dreadful thing to happen to you all year but chances are no one has even noticed it.

3. Feel good, look good. Be healthy. Eat well and exercise. If you feel like you're in shape, you will ooze confidence.

'All you need in this life are ignorance and confidence; then success is sure.'
MARK TWAIN

4. A new outfit/haircut/lip gloss can do wonders for your confidence levels. Treat yourself before an important date.

5. It's not about what you've got but what people think you've got. So if you feel your chest is a tad too flat, invest in a Wonderbra. If your lips are not plump enough then use some lipliner to accentuate them.

Another good trick is to remain slightly mysterious. If you're confident enough, don't let it all hang out on the first date. And don't fall into that trap of drinking too much and discussing what you did and didn't like about sex with your ex boyfriend. There won't be much left to the imagination after that conversation. Remember the old saying: fantasy is often better than reality. Don't give too much away.

So be confident and mysterious. If you feel suddenly insignificant then cast your mind back to your vast list of achievements and plus points. And remember, the person you're talking to is probably not as confident as they are pretending to be either...

'No one can make you feel inferior without your consent.'
ELEANOR ROOSEVELT

How did it go?

Q   **What sort of goals are you talking about?**

A   *I am talking about small things like doing fifty pelvic floor exercises every day, exfoliating three times a week or cleaning out your wardrobe. These are not things that one can fail at as they are not serious but they keep your mind focused on improving you.*

Q   **I can't stop worrying about how I look. Any tips?**

A   *Above all do not fidget. Confident and sexy people do not fidget: they don't need to because they know everything is as it should be. However much you want to whip out that mirror to check your lipstick, hair, false eyelashes – don't. How is anyone going to believe you are the supreme sexual god or goddess of the universe if you don't believe it yourself?*

15

Keep an eye on your eyebrows

Eyebrows can take years off you if you shape them right. Here's how to do it without looking constantly surprised.

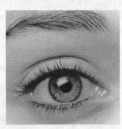

An untamed monobrow is great if you're going for the Frida Kahlo look, but if you want to look groomed, elegant and more alert and wide-eyed, it's time to pay your brows some attention.

Think of eyebrow-shaping as treating yourself to an upper facelift on the cheap. Trim, neat, naturally ascending arched brows can make your eyes appear bigger and give you a more youthful appearance. If your brows are wild, tousled, virgin territory, you're missing a key beauty trick.

So, where do you start? There are various different brow-defining options, depending on what you want to achieve. If you've recently gone lighter or darker and don't want your eyebrows to give you away, you can try tinting, which really ought to be done by a beautician. Then there's the choice between plucking, waxing or even threading. Threading is a wonderful Middle Eastern technique that involves tiny intertwined threads being rubbed gently over the eyebrow hairs. This

Here's an idea for you...

Give yourself a facial workout to help tone your facial muscles and delay the ageing process. Stand in front of the mirror daily and raise your eyebrows as high as possible and simultaneously open your eyes as wide as you can. Slowly lower your eyebrows and relax. Repeat this five times.

stings slightly, but threading doesn't leave a red mark and some find it's the least painful option. Most salon eyebrow shaping involves a bit of waxing, then tidying up with a pair of tweezers.

If you're going to splurge on a visit to the beautician, some would say that eyebrow shaping is the treatment to have done. It doesn't cost the earth, but it's a fabulous investment. If you have your brows shaped just two or three times yearly, you'll have a template to follow at home. All you need to do is simply 'tidy' them once or twice a week with a pair of tweezers.

HOME PLUCKING: THE RULES

If you choose to go it alone, tread carefully. You can make some pretty awful mistakes with eyebrows and end up looking permanently surprised, shifty or botoxed to within an inch of your life. Always pluck in a good light and invest in a magnifying mirror.

- Start by brushing your eyebrows, using an eyebrow brush or small, soft toothbrush. Then trim any long hairs with nail scissors.
- Aim for a natural, gently curving arch, thicker in the inner corner of the eye and tapering out over your brow bone. Focus on accentuating this natural curve by tidying up around it, above (forget that old myth, you *can* pluck above the brow) and below.

- Each eyebrow should start directly above the corner of the eye and should be the same width as your eye. Hold a pencil vertically along the side of your nose and remove any wild or stray hairs on the bridge of your nose beyond the pencil with a pair of tweezers.

- Then, to see where your eyebrow should end, hold the pencil diagonally from your nostril to the end of your eye and pluck anything below the pencil to open up your eyes and to avoid looking drowsy.

- Then work on the natural arch. To find the highest part of the arch, imagine drawing a line from the outer edge of your iris right up to your browline. That should be the highest point of your eyebrow arch. Tweeze any hairs underneath that arch. Don't go mad though. Natural is always better.

- If you want a fuller look, try brushing your brows sideways with your little toothbrush or eyebrow brush. Or slick them down using Vaseline or a bit of moisturiser. You can buy eyebrow gel, but it's not vital unless you have very unruly eyebrows. Slicked eyebrows do make you look instantly groomed, though, so it's worth experimenting with gels.

'Elegance is innate.... It has nothing to do with being well-dressed.'
DIANA VREELAND

Defining idea...

How did
it go?

Q   **It's so painful! Any tips on plucking without needing a general anaesthetic?**

A   *Either tackle your eyebrows after a bath when your pores are slightly open or after placing a warm damp flannel over your forehead. And the plucking itself will be easier if you pull the skin as taut as you can. Always pluck in the direction the hairs grow to minimise the sting and use ice cubes to reduce redness and soothe the burn after the job is done.*

Q   **Can you overpluck and end up totally eyebrow-less?**

A   *Yes. Brows get thinner and sparser with age and continuous overplucking doesn't help. Also, if you pluck hairs enough, they'll eventually stop growing completely. So, do try not to go mad with the tweezers!*

Q   **I've got an eyebrow pencil, but how do I know when or even whether I need to use it?**

A   *If your brows are even and not patchy you won't actually need one. However, if you've overplucked and need to 'restore' your eyebrow, then an eyebrow pencil will do the trick. Avoid that obvious 'drawn on' look though and use a blend of pencil and eyeshadow. Use a shade as close as possible or slightly darker than your hair colour and apply it with a little brush. But don't go too dark or it'll look theatrical!*

16

Love the skin you're in

Coping with those hilarious skin changes during pregnancy.
Can you avoid stretch marks?

Glowing skin or spotty as a teenager?
The hormonal changes you experience during
pregnancy can make some odd things happen to
your skin, but there are simple remedies.

FACIAL SPOTS

You may find that your skin breaks out more in pregnancy, despite all that healthy eating and clean living! This is because oil (sebum) production increases during pregnancy. Your skin produces sebum in order to keep it soft and supple. The sudden increase can make spots appear, particularly in the last trimester – a little like they do before a period. You may have noticed that the tiny oil glands ('Montgomery's tubercles') around your nipples have become bigger. This helps protect your nipples and stops them from drying out during breastfeeding. Things will return to normal after delivery.

To deal with the extra sebum, use gentle, hypoallergenic products to step up your skincare routine. Drink lots of water, and eat plenty of foods containing vitamin B6

Here's an idea for you...

Make yourself a gentle facial scrub from fine oatmeal from a health food shop mixed with honey and a little water. Smooth it onto your skin and make circular motions with your fingers before washing it off with cotton wool and tepid water. If you can bear it, splash your face with cold water to close your pores after you have finished. Avoid the use of harsh exfoliants.

such as wholegrain cereals and breads, potatoes, bananas and peanut butter. Vitamin B6 helps to control hormonally induced skin problems. Don't be tempted to take supplements unless you have consulted your doctor. On the subject of medication, do *not* take any of the anti-acne prescription drugs such as Accutane and Retin-A during pregnancy: they carry a high risk of causing birth defects.

SWEATY BETTY

When you are pregnant, you sweat more. You are also heavier than you were pre-pregnancy, and this can make you puffy in places. The upshot of this may be sweat rash under your boobs and in your groin. This is uncomfortable – and difficult to shift, once it occurs. Treat sweat rashes by bathing the area in cool water. You can also apply a sprinkling of cornflour to reduce chafing.

ITCHY!

As your belly and breasts grow, and your skin stretches, you may feel generalised itching. Make your showers and baths warm rather than hot – really hot baths that raise your temperature are not good for your baby anyway. Only use mild soap or bath gel and use a moisturizer regularly. Applying that could be a fun job for the boys...

If your skin is really itchy, dissolve a cup of bicarbonate of soda in your bath for a soothing soak. If the itching is *really* bad, or you have a persistent rash, contact your healthcare provider for a check up.

DREADED STRETCH MARKS OR HONOURABLE SCARS?

Stretch marks are the source of many a joke, but they are something women really dread. And yes, I have some. But then again, so do many bodybuilders, apparently. My dad calls them honourable scars, but he is a bit of a charmer. Check out your mum if you are worried about stretch marks. They run in the family.

Stretch marks are small tears made in response to the pulling and stretching your poor dermis undergoes as you expand. Sadly, the jury is still out as to whether any of the (expensive) lotions and potions available are effective. If it makes you feel better, have a go – you have nothing to lose, and it's a great excuse to make your partner give you a lovely rub down with Shea butter. A win–win situation, I'd say.

If you do get stretch marks, try not to worry. They start off red, but fade to silver.

WHO'S BEEN PAINTING ON MY BELLY?

You may wake up one day to find you have a dark line running from your pubes up to your belly button. No, your partner hasn't been busy with the magic markers; it's another of nature's little jokes. The line is called the linea nigra, found more often in women with darker skin and hair. Before you became pregnant, you had an unnoticeable line in the same place. When you are pregnant, you produce more melanin and that causes the line to darken. It usually disappears again after the birth.

> *'Some cultures believe the linea nigra is the result of a high concentration of "chi". The "chi" energy is working intensely to create a new life force – your baby – and the linea nigra is the external manifestation of that energy working!'*
> PHOEBE JACKSON, doula

Defining idea...

65

How did it go?

Q **I had a baby six weeks ago, but the brown line down the middle of my belly – which my midwife assured me would disappear – is still there! Why?**

A *It often takes a few months for all of the hormones that have been raging round your body to settle to their pre-pregnancy levels. Once they have gone, the line will fade. Since the line appears as a result of the production of melanin, you may want to keep your tummy hidden from the sun until the line has faded. Or like me, four babies later, you may want to keep your belly hidden. Period.*

Q **I have developed some dark patches on my face that my mum has called a 'butterfly mask'. To me it looks more like a tea stain! How can I get rid of it?**

A *The patches are the 'mask of pregnancy', or melasma, a dark patch of skin that develops sometimes on the cheeks, upper lip and forehead of a pregnant woman. It is common, and doctors believe it may be caused by the action of the hormone oestrogen combined with exposure to sunlight. It will fade after the birth of your baby, and you may want to hasten fading by applying a natural face mask made from kaolin powder mixed with lemon juice and natural yoghurt. Just watch out for wasps!*

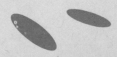

17

Sex up your legs

How to slim, tone, smooth, soften and flatter them, whatever their shape.

Nothing will produce more wolf whistles than a pair of slim, shapely legs. If you're not convinced, just pull on some hot pants and head to your nearest building site now!

Sadly, not everyone is as forgiving as builders when it comes to legs. We're our own worst critics, in fact. But if you keep them smooth, toned, bronzed and moisturised, your legs will take you a lot further in life than from A to B.

LONG AND LEAN

If your legs are carrying extra weight, you'll transform them just by shifting some pounds with a low-fat, low-calorie diet. A combination of cardiovascular and resistance exercise is the best way to reduce overall body fat; aim for three thirty-minute cardio sessions such as running, rowing or cycling, and three total body-resistance workouts a week. You'll need to include dynamic work such as squats, lunges and step-ups in your resistance workout. All of these can be done in the comfort of your home and will improve the muscular tone of your legs. Your

Here's an idea for you...

Be clever with tights. Black opaques make legs svelte and go with pretty much everything. Choose tights with vertical stripes to make your legs look longer and leaner. Fishnets can also look fantastic, but stick to more flattering narrow weaves and dark colours. Avoid red or white like the plague and don't team tights with minis unless you're a lady of the night.

hamstring muscles will need work too; they tend to be weaker and so have a tendency to display the delightful traits of cellulite more than other areas. Uphill walking is great for hamstrings. If you're a gym member, sign up for classes such as body pump and body conditioning, and try dance-based classes such as cardio funk. Pilates and yoga are also great for sculpting long, lean leg muscles.

Try the following key exercises. Aim to do three sets of each exercise, three times a week.

THIGH, BUM AND CALF FIRMERS

Straight leg lunge

Stand on a step and then take a large stride off it, extending one leg back behind you. Your front knee should be over your front ankle and the back leg should be long with a slight bend at the knee. Keep the back knee and heel off the floor. Contract through your tummy muscles as you lift yourself back up to a straight position. Change legs. Do twelve on each leg, building up to three sets.

THIGH TONERS

Squats

Stand with your feet wider than hip-width
apart, with your toes and knees pointing out at
forty-five degrees and your hands on your thighs. Pull up through your tummy
muscles. Bend your knees, lowering your torso towards the floor. Keep the weight
on your heels, and your spine in neutral position with your tailbone pointing down
as you lower. Draw your weight onto one leg as you drag the other towards it. Use
your inner thighs to draw your legs together. Draw your legs apart and repeat on
the other side. Repeat twelve to fifteen times on each leg, again building up to
three sets.

SMOOTH AND SOFT

For this you need to exfoliate regularly using a loofah, body brush or exfoliating
mitt. Try body-brushing every morning before your shower or bath; use a brush
with natural fibres and gently brush upwards towards the heart in long, sweeping
motions. Exfoliators are great for softening the hard skin on knees too. Keep legs
well moisturised at all times; creams and lotions help plump up the upper layer of
skin and make it look softer, smoother and younger.

*'I have flabby thighs, but
fortunately my stomach
covers them.'*
JOAN RIVERS

Defining
idea...

BRONZED

A tan will automatically give the impression of longer, slimmer, more even-textured legs. Fake tan is the best way to get a safe year-round tan. Always exfoliate first and massage in a light moisturiser before applying your tanning product. Don't overdo your heels or knees though, as these areas tend to get patchy.

SHIMMERY

Rubbing body oil into your legs will make them shimmer seductively and look particularly gorgeous over tanned skin. Even olive, sunflower or almond oil will do the trick.

Defining idea...

'Darling, the legs aren't so beautiful, I just know what to do with them.'
MARLENE DIETRICH

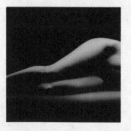
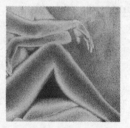
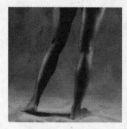

Q   What's the best way to remove leg hair?

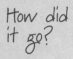

A   *It depends how hirsute you are. It also depends on your pain threshold. Waxing involves plucking the hairs from below the surface, so the results last about two to three weeks longer than shaving or using a depilatory cream. Chemical depilatories break down the protein structure of the hairs and are wiped off. If your skin is sensitive, always test a small area first. The hair that re-grows won't feel as rough and bristly as after shaving, plus it takes longer to reappear. If you're shaving always wet the area with a shaving gel or cream, or even a moisturiser. This way you're less likely to nick yourself and you'll get a closer shave because hair absorbs water, making it stiffer and easier to cut. Always moisturise after shaving.*

Q   I dread summer as my legs weren't made for shorts. What's the most flattering shape?

A   *You can lengthen short legs with slightly flared 'short' shorts. Or try shorts that just skim your mid thighs. Avoid wearing socks and trainers if your legs are short and pudgy; stick to sandals with a bit of a heel to create a longer expanse of leg. As for skirts, A-line is the best cut, just below the knees. When buying skirts, trousers and shorts, never choose a cut that stops in the thickest part of your leg, whether that's your thighs, knees or calves. Again, a heel always makes a leg look slimmer, so invest in some comfortable kitten heels. Leggings don't look good on anyone over eight (that goes for both age and stones).*

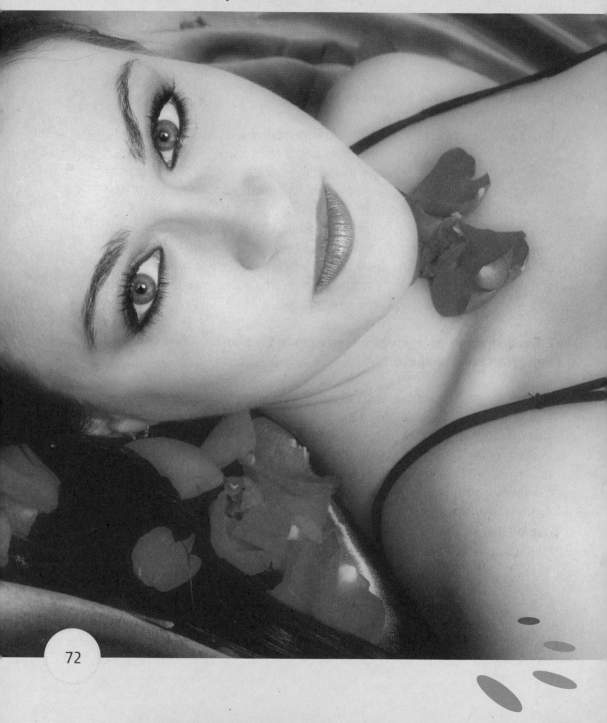

18

Sexy style

Image, style, look. Call it what you want, but you need to define it. Your style is something that is all about you.

You can change things, add accessories, lose weight, put on more lipstick but unless you ooze your own personal style, it won't make much difference to your sex appeal.

A friend of mine was recently extremely irritated with her husband. They have been married for five years and he won't let her wear her old leggings around the house. 'I know they're not the most attractive item of clothing I have,' she says. 'But they're so comfortable and I love them. He says they look awful and he doesn't want to see me in them.' Some of you might say that's unreasonable, but I have begun to side with the husband in this argument. My friend would never have worn her old leggings on their first date. So why lose your sexy style just because you're married? Surely being married is even more reason to make an effort, unless you want your husband to start looking for sexy stylish women elsewhere. Sexy style is something that should stay with you for ever, your own intangible look and image; leggings are for those rare moments alone, or with other girlfriends, who also have bits of comfort clothing they're longing to wear.

Here's an idea for you...

Transparent blouses are wonderfully sexy and no matter how little you like the idea there's a way to wear see-through without showing a thing. Fabric technology allows wispy fabrics that when you try them give just a hazy idea of what might be underneath. But if that's still too much, wear a jacket over it so there's only a glimpse of what's underneath. Alternatively a glimpse of lace works wonders.

So what style will you go for today? There are three classic looks that work well – romantic (flowing skirts), flirtatious (tight, short) and erotic (gorgeous clinging fabrics, seriously grown up). Obviously the image you choose is determined by where you are going and what you're going to be doing. It would be daft to show up for a walk on the beach with your latest paramour wearing a leather skirt and stilettos. If it's a simple style you're after try a pretty floral dress (or jeans if you're a bloke), chinos and T-shirt, a flowing skirt and a cashmere jumper, and go for soft colours such as beige, light blue or rose.

For a first date where there will be plenty of flirting going on, dress accordingly; a low-cut top or a short skirt (but never both together), go for warm, passionate colours like red, and remember your choice of underwear is crucial.

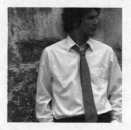
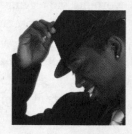

The vampy, flirtatious look is really not the one for a first date. You could come across as cheap and tarty, which he might think is ideal for that night but won't be any good for your long-term prospects. Unless of course you're just after a hugely erotic one-night stand, in which case, go for it. If you do want to dress in a way that guarantees he'll want to sleep with you then of course leather is good (preferably black), animal prints are also pretty effective and anything seriously short and figure hugging. Lots of cleavage (if you don't have it, fake it), zips in strategic places and lace-up tops.

Remember you are in control of the image you want to portray and the signals you want to send out to your date. Don't make them the wrong ones by either going over the top or showing up looking like a maiden aunt, though some men may even get off on that look. Best not to risk it though.

> *'Penguins mate for life. Which doesn't exactly surprise me that much 'cause they all look alike – it's not like they're gonna meet a better looking penguin some day.'*
> ELLEN DEGENERES, comedian

Defining idea...

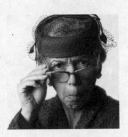

How did it go?

Q   Are you saying I need to look hot the whole time? How about just relaxing for a change?

A   *Of course you can relax, but do it stylishly. There's nothing uncomfortable about a cashmere jumper or a chic T-shirt and pair of chinos. There is even some rather sexy and stylish house-wear clothing around these days which is a great alternative to jammies or leggings.*

Q   What about make-up?

A   *Make-up is crucial. Your make-up should reflect your clothes. Do not mix a summery pink cashmere top and flowing skirt with the red lips look. Instead go for a little pale lip gloss. The little black dress can look great with thick, black eyelashes and red lips. Obviously make-up depends very much on your complexion and colouring. Get professional advice if you're not sure. Any Clarins counter (the earthly equivalent of heaven) will help. Don't forget that scent is important, and try to match your fragrance to your image. Some classics go with anything but you don't want to send out contradicting messages so take care.*

19

On the shelf

Cellulite creams abound. But what works, what doesn't and what's really worth the money?

There's no denying the placebo effect of using cellulite creams — there's nothing like rubbing on pricey, sweet-smelling, beautifully packaged unguents to make you feel you're spoiling yourself.

Well, do they work? You might be seduced into thinking so. These days many products are impressively endorsed by various scientific studies, many of which claim that testers lost inches and pounds after using said unguent for a period of time.

But if you're hoping for a miracle in a bottle, you still have a long wait. Cellulite creams alone, however impressive, aren't likely to transform fleshy, saggy buttocks into a nectarine-firm bottom.

But they may certainly help. Cellulite creams can hydrate your skin, so if your thighs and bottom have been neglected, rubbing on a cream will add moisture to the area and help plump up the skin. Big difference already.

Here's an idea for you... **Short on pennies? Try natural olive or grapeseed oil; you can buy them over the counter at chemists for next to nothing. Gentle enough for newborn babies, they're unlikely to cause reactions and are great for massage or for all over moisturising.**

Many cellulite creams also contain temporary toning ingredients, which help improve skin texture; the effects can be pretty immediate but are temporary – good for a hot date, beach day, black dress occasion, that sort of thing.

But the longer-lasting effects come down to a pot-pourri of active ingredients, which do anything from boost metabolism, facilitate cell turnover, help shed water, even break down fat.

Take *caffeine*, a common and effective ingredient in many anti-cellulite formulations. It's thought to encourage the metabolism of fats, and help drain accumulated fluids in your fat cells, and boost your circulation. It's also toning.

Another key ingredient used in the more effective anti-cellulite creams is *retinol*. It's a derivative of vitamin A that has been found to increase skin renewal and boost the production of collagen. Often found in face cream, it can improve the elasticity of the skin on your nether regions too. RoC's retinol-based product has many devotees, who claim to have lost inches and firmed up significantly using the formulation twice daily.

Another cellulite-busting ingredient is *aminophylline*, which is thought by some experts to enter the bloodstream and actually break down fat in the cells. One study found women using aminophylline cream lost as much as 8 mm from their thighs. Another study showed impressive results with *aminophylline*, although it was used alongside a calorie-reduced diet and daily exercise too.

Exfoliating ingredients such as *alpha-hydroxy acids* (AHAs) are often used in the latest cellulite-busting products. AHAs are found in plants (citrus fruits and apples) and are used in skin products to help remove dead skin cells, thereby promoting the turnover of new cells. Thus far research has found the effects on cellulitey areas tend to be temporary, rather than permanent, but watch this space.

'I will buy any cream, cosmetic, or elixir from a woman with a European accent.'
ERMA BOMBECK, humorist

Defining idea...

Natural ingredients

Most treatment creams are a combination of cutting-edge technology alongside tried and trusted natural or herbal ingredients. Here are a few to look out for:

■ **Gingko biloba** can stimulate your circulation and boost blood flow. It's a strong antioxidant, so it may help slow down the ageing process and help fight the free radicals that can cause your skin to age.

■ **Gotu kola**. This herb is thought to enhance the production of collagen. It's good for circulation and also has diuretic qualities. It's been found to help heal wounds and burns, so has positive effects on skin tissue.

■ **Guarana** is a natural stimulant with a strong diuretic action. This seed is thought to help boost metabolism, and also has antioxidant qualities.

■ **Horse chestnut** can help reduce water retention, boost circulation and increase blood flow to the skin.

- **Butcher's broom** is a plant extract with a diuretic action and may help boost circulation.

- **Ivy** has been found to help boost the circulation. It also has astringent properties, which may have a temporary toning effect on cellulite.

- **Marine extracts** such as carrageenan and alginic acid can help draw water into the skin which may help make cellulite look less obvious by filling in the dimples.

- **Co-enzyme Q10** is a powerful antioxidant thought to help beat cellulite by helping build collagen, thereby countering skin sagginess.

Q **I've been using this cream day and night for a week, but can't yet see any results yet. Am I doing it right?**

How did it go?

A *Have you read the packet? Many cellulite formulations are designed to be used alongside regular exercise and a low-fat healthy diet, and ideally applied twice daily using a five-minute self-massage technique, so the cream itself is just one prong in your attack. Most manufacturers also state the product needs to be used for at least thirty days before you see results. Also, bear in mind the results may be subtle rather than miraculous.*

Q **Are those massagers that come with the product any good?**

A *Depends. They're said to help you stimulate the area, and massage is believed to boost circulation and lymph drainage. Avoid rubbing over-zealously though; it can damage the tissue and make matters worse. Manipulating your cellulitey areas with a brush or loofah or special massager may certainly have an exfoliating effect, which can improve the texture of the skin instantly.*

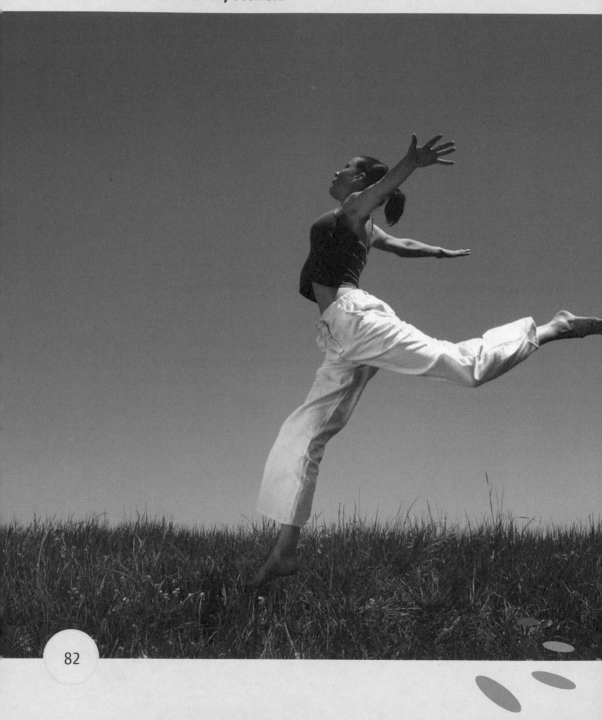

20

Lighten up

Joie de vivre radiates outwards, which is why happy people are more attractive. Here's how to get your sparkle back.

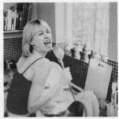

You only have to read the personal ads to see what women believe makes them attractive to the opposite sex. Youth and good looks, basically. But that's not the whole picture.

Women are brought up to believe that physical characteristics rather than wit or a sense of optimism determine our attractiveness. We can't be expected to both look decorative *and* tell jokes, surely? But let's face it, there's something appealing and uplifting about being around someone who's optimistic, bright and funny.

For a start, a breezy, happy attitude and a good sense of humour can reduce stressful situations, diffuse tension, build bridges, heal relationships and make those around us feel happier too. So, it's little wonder that someone who makes us laugh or laughs with us is going to appear attractive.

Having fun is also really good for you. A good laugh is like having an internal workout, as laughter can produce feel-good chemicals and ones that boost our

Here's an idea for you... Get a sheet of paper and list your reasons to be happy. Start with today's events then cover life in general. Write down anything at all that puts a smile on your face or a warm glow in your belly such as a fantastic family, a great job or even a bargain pair of shoes.

immune system. Apparently a good laugh can reduce the levels of the stress hormone in your blood by 30% and it can help burn calories (as many as 500 calories per hour), plus when we laugh we release the natural pain-relaxant endorphin, which is also released during exercise. And after a good laughter session your heart rate and blood pressure drop, your muscles relax and you breathe more deeply.

A strong wit can make a plain woman beautiful. For a start, the ability to tell jokes and make smart, witty asides will make you look both clever and confident, and as we all well know, confidence is hugely seductive. Humour also enables you to laugh at your own foibles, find a funny side to embarrassing situations and find the silver lining to setbacks.

So, what if you're simply not an 'up' person. Will a bit of impromptu goose-stepping or crazy-wig wearing do the trick? Er, no. You don't have to be a laugh-a-minute comedienne to have *joie de vivre*. It's not about having an ability to get people rolling in the aisles. The key is to be able to have fun, be optimistic and see the best side of everything. A humorous attitude can help us to see life from a positive perspective and face problems with renewed ability and hope. And that's infectious.

If you've lost that sparkle, try these approaches:

- Spend time with children. They know how to have fun.
- Play games in the park, go to a theme park, have a girly tea party, that sort of thing.
- Look back at your last crisis. Can you find a funny side to it?
- Dig out old photos and look at the hairdos, guaranteed to put a smile on your face (well, everyone else's hairdo will).
- Start savouring the pleasurable things in life. Try a new hobby, go on a shopping spree or get back to nature. Step out of your usual routine to find fun, laughter and adventure. Surround yourself with gorgeous things and your funniest friends.
- Get lots of fresh air. Run about, get soaked in a downpour, head for the coast and experience a sea storm, get up early and watch the sunrise, walk around barefoot, etc.
- Be your own therapist and try to write or retell your most painful or difficult moments with humour (focus on any break-ups or the time you got the sack as opposed to car crashes or life-threatening operations). Experts say this can be a good way to exorcise demons and flex those optimism muscles.

'An inordinate passion for pleasure is the secret of remaining young.'
OSCAR WILDE

Defining idea...

85

How did it go?

Q **I'm feeling a bit flat and I know it shows. Is there any way to snap out of it?**

A *Not instantly, but a little comedy one evening should help. Humour is like a muscle; you need to exercise it. Get a stash of funny videos and savour the innuendos. Laugh and cry. Think of it as a personality workout. Seek out comic books, TV shows and films that mirror your personal trauma.*

Q **How can I look more confident and 'up'?**

A *Just smile more, even if you don't feel like it. Smiling faces are always rated more attractive than non-smiling ones. Remember that a genuine smile goes to your eyes, so make sure it's a crinkly-eye one rather than a lower-face-only 'politician' smile.*

Q **I've got a scary presentation and want to look my best. Any tips?**

A *Brush up your repartee. A few funny lines or wisecracks can make people warm to you, so work on your own collection of amusing anecdotes or one-liners and use them to pepper your script. Practise them in front of the mirror, till they're smooth and seamless.*

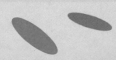

21

Beauty and the breast

All the magazines are full of images of skinny women with tiny waists and thin faces. Being a size 10 is old hat. Now we should aspire to be a size 6.

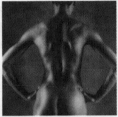

It's crazy. Because one thing is for sure. The old adage that men like something they can get hold of still stands.

If you are voluptuous, use it, play to your advantage. Wear clothes that accentuate your chest and hips, thus making your waist look thinner. Think classic movie star hourglass figure. A friend of mine fluctuates between a size 12 and 14. She is very pretty but lacked confidence as she thought she was too fat. She spent years going on awful diets that made her feel dreadful. Still her body shape remained the same. 'One day I was walking home from work, it was sunny and I was wearing a T-shirt and long flowing skirt. My hair was loose and I was feeling quite chirpy,' she says. 'A total stranger came up to me and gave me a rose. He told me he had been carrying it the whole day looking for a woman that epitomised his ideal to present it to. For the first time ever it occurred to me that I was sexy just the way I am.'

Here's an idea for you...

If you are toned you will never look out of shape, no matter how voluptuous you are. You should do sit-ups, press-ups and bottom clenches every day. Hone those beautiful curves until they are irresistibly perfect.

The fact that Marilyn Monroe was a size 14 has often been quoted. The first time I heard it, I couldn't believe it. I thought it was impossible that a sex symbol could be so, well, large. In fact if you watch her wiggling down the platform in the film *Some Like it Hot*, you can see she really does have what you might call child-bearing hips. But there's no denying that she is one of the sexiest film stars of all time.

So the lesson is, if you've got it, flaunt it. Wear tops that accentuate your cleavage and wear bras that make the best of your breasts. If you are short then avoid horizontal stripes as they will accentuate your size; go for vertical stripes or plain colours. Choose clothes and colours that exaggerate your femininity; long flowing dresses, pastel colours, lace (with a hint of cleavage showing of course). If you worry about your bottom being too big, wear loose trousers with side fastenings. These flatten your tummy and minimise your bum.

The skinny ideal that we're all supposed to aspire to is only something propagated by fashion designers and marketing forces, according to a website which celebrates the hourglass figure. It goes on to say that the hourglass or pear-shaped female form has been idolised for centuries.

Less than 3 per cent of American women are the size of the models that grace the front covers of all the magazines. So 97 per cent of them are unattractive are they? That means an awful lot of so-called unattractive women are getting married, laid, falling in love, having children every day. Go figure. It's got to be the magazines that have got it wrong.

'I know that there are nights when I have power. When I put on something and walk in somewhere and if there is a man who doesn't look at me, it's because he's gay.'
KATHLEEN TURNER, actor

Defining idea...

The other good news is that being slightly plump makes you look younger. Skinny women have more lines. The English poet John Dryden said: 'I am resolved to grow fat and look young at 40, and then slip out of the world with the first wrinkle and the reputation of five-and-twenty.' That's the poetic way of stating the unavoidable truth: as she grows older a woman has to make a choice between her face and her bum. She can't keep both in the same condition as when she was 20.

For that reason, Dr Jean-Louis Sebagh, one of Europe's leading beauticians and botox experts, recommends that women over 35 should not try to lose weight.

How did it go?

Q **I can't bear the size of my breasts. They are vast. I feel so embarrassed about them. What can I do to hide them?**

A *Speaking as a girl whose highlight in life was finding that at seven months pregnant my tits had gone from an A cup to a D cup, I can't really muster up much sympathy for your particular problem. I suppose we all want what we haven't got, but there is no getting away from the fact that men LOVE big tits. I don't know why, maybe it's a mummy thing, but they just do. OK, so there are things you can do to lessen your curves, bras you can buy and certain colours and cuts of clothes that will diminish the effect, but why bother? Be proud of your chest. Carry it well, don't slouch and try to hide it. Women all over the world will be insanely jealous and men will be falling over themselves to please you.*

Q **This is all very well. But inside every fat woman isn't there a skinny-woman wanting to get out?**

A *If you're really unhappy about your size then you can do something about it. Go on a detox for a week (no dairy, no wheat, no sugar) and see how much excess weight comes off. But don't blame me if your boyfriend starts complaining.*

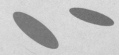

22

Lose 10 lb without dieting

**Dress cleverly – in shades, cuts and styles to suit you. It's
the simplest way to look slimmer and more shapely.**

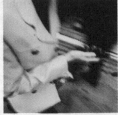

I rarely used to dress in anything other
than black, even at the type of events
that begged for the most feminine florals and
pastel chiffon. I mistakenly believed that black
made me look barely-there thin.

Now it's true that black can undoubtedly look supremely elegant. In fact, the longer
the streak you create, the better. Dark colours certainly can minimise the bulges,
but it's not the only sartorial route to a more slender you. Besides, black can also be
dreary and draining. And if you get it ever so slightly wrong at functions, you'll have
half a dozen coats flung at you or be asked for another vol-au-vent, both of which,
when you're aiming for willowy Eva Herzigova-esque grandeur, will negate the joys
of a slightly smaller arse. Instead, be inventive and follow these guidelines:

■ Minimise bulges by sticking to pretty much any colour. Dark colours are obviously
the most flattering, but in summer you can still create the illusion of being longer
and leaner if you're dressed head to foot in the same shade, even white.

Here's an
idea for
you...

Colour experts say white, silver and mother of pearl are 'eternally feminine' because they're associated with the moon, stars and sea. Remember that luminous uber-gown that Nicole Kidman wore to the Oscars a few years ago? Investing in striking silver or pearl jewellery is the easiest way to wear these colours. Alternatively, tap into your inner goddess with a soft shell-pink wrap and mother-of-pearl make-up that will look particularly great against a tan. Light colours close to your face can reflect light and take years off you, too.

- Ignore size tags when you're shopping. Don't buy the snug size 10 just because that's your usual size. You can lose pounds by wearing slightly looser clothes that skim over bumps and hang flatteringly.

- Where possible, choose lined clothes. They won't hug you so unforgivingly. Lined trousers are a godsend, particularly in summer, as they drop crisply, however hot and sweaty you are beneath.

- Invest in an A-line skirt. These flatter almost everyone because they don't cling to your curves but do minimise your bottom. The best length is on or just below the knee, and if you team it with knee-length boots you can disguise thick legs and hefty unfeminine thighs. In the summer, a light-coloured skirt can look great with suede or denim boots.

- Don't be afraid of hipster jeans. They may seem the preserve of nubile girly band members, but they can be really flattering whatever your age as they create the illusion of smaller hips. Keep a close eye on the flesh overhang, however, which can ruin the effect, and if possible stick to the boot-leg cut, which is flattering as it makes your legs look longer and slimmer.

- Always wear a heel, however slight. Even very tall women can get away with tiny tapering heels. The extra inch or two will add length and can make you more aware of your posture.

- Stick to textured fabrics, which can help to 'break up' flesh. Think linen, wool or even crinkled man-made fabrics.

- Disguise a big bust with V-necks and low scoop necks. Avoid slash necks and halter necks altogether as they make women look bulky.

- Always choose trousers with hems long enough to skim the tip of a boot or shoe. They may feel too long, but they'll immediately draw the eye down, giving the impression of a longer, leaner leg. Also, avoid tapered trousers, clam diggers and pedal pushers, which make almost everyone's thighs look bigger and legs look shorter and squatter.

- Investing in good lingerie can knock pounds off you. So, go for well-fitting bras with uplift and knickers that flatten in the right places. With bras, aim to banish seams, puckering and surplus flesh bursting out of cups (unless that's what you're aiming for).

'I have always said that the best clothes are invisible...they make you notice the person.'
KATHARINE HAMNETT

Defining idea...

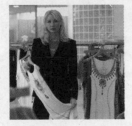
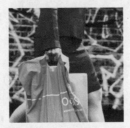

93

How did it go?

Q   **I don't have a clothing allowance for a new wardrobe! Any tips?**

A   *Take a good look at your present collection and sift mercilessly. Hang clothes of the same colour together so you can see what you're working with and it's easier to co-ordinate. If possible, buy just a few key items from the list above. I suggest you enlist the help of an honest but well-meaning friend who will read the above rules and help you apply them before your next sortie.*

Q   **Do you have any useful tips for buying flattering jackets?**

A   *Lined, tailored, single-breasted jackets are a great investment if you're big busted, as they make you look neater. And bear in mind that a jacket that just skims your bottom will disguise a big bottom far better than a short, over-fitted jacket will.*

23

Tricks of the trade

It's finally happened, the date you have been waiting for for six months is on. The man of your dreams is going to meet you, just you, for a totally romantic time and it's going to happen...tonight.

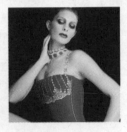

Help. You still can't get into those trousers you swore you would slim your way into a year ago. Your waistline is way over its ideal and you have three hours to change it.

No point in dieting now. Reach for those pants of steel. Remember Bridget Jones? These miracle workers basically compress your flesh and reduce your waistline. You can get those that reach down to your thighs as well. They come in all shapes and sizes with reassuring names like 'body slimmers' and 'hi-waist busters'. They can be found on the web and in department stores. 'Quite miraculously, these can – and do – take a couple of inches off your waist and stop you looking like you're four months pregnant,' says India Knight in her book *The Shops*, 'without the excess flesh making a reappearance elsewhere.'

95

Here's an idea for you...

The cosmetics counter can also help. Fake tan, firming and lifting serums and exfoliators can all make a contribution. Try those that offer an instant toning effect. Rub them on any skin that is on show and watch it glow.

Another, less restricting option is tights. Lots of retailers sell ranges of slimming tights, which are great but take an age to peel off due to their compressing nature. (Pants of steel are not easy to take off either, you'll need a very determined date to get round them. In short, these are bits of underwear to wear to impress as opposed to seduce.)

One thing that can be both slimming and seductive is a corset. I once had a Vivienne Westwood corset which had the most amazing effect on my (non-existent) tits. As a result I felt incredibly sexy wearing it, it was also very slimming on the waist, although when I last tried it on (three children and fifteen years later) the waist was a bit too high to be really flattering so it's now in the dressing-up box. I have now moved on to Chantal Thomass's corsets. My particular favourite is leopard skin (what mid-life crisis?). Her products are available in large department stores and other lingerie outlets worldwide. A corset will set you back around £120 (€175) but it's worth it purely for the effect it has on your waist and breasts. Wear it with jeans and a cashmere cardigan to achieve the greatest sexy impact.

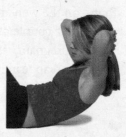

Don't forget the top half, too. Minimising bras can contribute to a svelte shape. This is not a garment I have ever had to wear but I gather from a friend who has that the problem is one of excess flesh squashed down by the bra turning up in strange places. My advice would be to ditch the minimising bra and strut your chest with pride. Men love boobs, there's no denying it. For those of you with little or no chest (like me) there is the maximising bra or Wonderbra. This is an essential piece of kit. It is worth spending proper money on this as cheap ones are rarely as effective.

Sexiness is all about confidence, and these little props will help you feel gorgeous, and boost your ego.

'Love is just a system for getting someone to call you darling after sex.'
JULIAN BARNES

Defining idea...

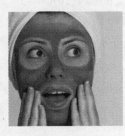
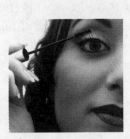

How did it go?

Q   **What is the point of wearing pants of steel when he's going to see what you really look like when he gets them off?**

A   *Fair point, but the image of you waltzing into the room looking serene and thin will stay with him for ever. Image is everything in the seduction game. The better you feel about the way you look the more you are going to ooze confidence and sexiness. I promise you it's worth a try, those pants of steel really do work wonders, and miraculously one can still breathe while wearing them. When it comes to undressing, dim the lights. In fact, turn them off!*

Q   **How about not eating anything at all the day of the date? Surely then I'll look thinner?**

A   *Possibly, but you might also get horribly drunk and light headed and fall over on your way to the loo. Not a good look. By all means don't stuff your face, eat in moderation and do not eat any garlic under any circumstances. Also be aware of foods that make you bloated (possibly some fruit and vegetables) and avoid them. Huge amounts of fizzy water will bloat you too. Avoiding fizzy drinks is an obvious tip, but that goes for all the time, not just before a date. Another thing to avoid is chewing gum which can make you feel bloated. Ideally eat something light like some lean meat or chicken before heading out to keep you from being ravenous but avoid enlarging your silhouette.*

24

Move that body

**Exercise has the potential to transform your body and do
wonders for your skin. And it's free!**

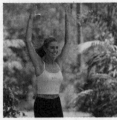

There's nothing to beat a post-workout
glow — the radiant skin and sparkling
eyes. Except perhaps the smug knowledge that
you've burnt calories and helped tone your wobbly
bits.

Like love, exercise is a drug. It can make you feel amazing and crap simultaneously.
Extraordinary things happen at a physiological level when you exercise, too. When
you start moving, endorphins – natural opiates – are released, which block your
body's pain receptors so you feel almost euphoric.

Exercise is great for your complexion, too, because it boosts blood circulation,
which gives your skin a healthy glow and helps draw out impurities. When you
exercise, a growth hormone is secreted into your body, which helps thicken and
firm up the skin and puts wrinkles on hold. Studies have shown that athletes' skin
is thicker and contains more collagen than other people's. The good news is that
even a small amount of exercise can make a major difference. The aim is to increase

Here's an idea for you...

Couch potatoes can turn an evening vegging in front of the TV into a workout by fidgeting more, which can apparently burn up to 800 calories a day. So make a point of shifting around every fifteen minutes – adjust your posture, roll your shoulders or change the way you cross your legs. The same goes for sitting at your desk or driving.

oxygen to the skin. At rest the average person takes in about 0.5 litres of air with every breath, but with exercise your air intake can increase to 4.5 litres per breath, which means a lot more oxygen is getting to your skin.

Experts say we should aim for a minimum of three twenty- to thirty-minute aerobic sessions per week, such as running, swimming, cycling, dancing or brisk walking. If possible, also try to add in three half-hour sessions of weight or resistance work, which increases muscle mass and can boost your body's metabolism and improve the way your body handles free radicals. These wreak havoc on your body, including your skin – so invest in some dumbbells or try walking or cycling uphill.

If you're new to exercise, don't rush it. Start small and be realistic about what you want to achieve. Don't declare you're going to lose a stone in two weeks, which would be neither healthy nor realistic. Instead, focus on an event, such as having to fit into a dress. Every week aim to do something, even if it's a twenty-minute stroll every other day. Make a list of what you're going to do each week and stick to it. And try to change your approach to exercise and think of it as a way to de-stress, energise and make your skin glow, not merely 'burning calories'.

Exercise may also make you more interesting! Studies have shown that long-distance exercise such as rowing, walking, running or swimming is good for creativity because while you're doing it your brain is 'set free'. Anything over ten minutes counts.

Try getting some friends on board. If you make a social event of your exercise, you're more likely to stick at it. In one recent study, people who made friends at their gym tended to exercise more often than people without gym buddies. If you're not a gym member, make dates to walk or exercise with a friend to help you keep on track.

'*A bear, however hard he tries, grows tubby without exercise.*'
WINNIE THE POOH

Defining idea...

If you're not a natural exerciser, the key is to think in terms of activities rather than workouts as activities will sound less like a chore. Swimming, hiking, cycling, walking or rollerblading are far more appealing than going to the gym. They're fun, burn calories and are great for sculpting thighs, bottoms and legs. Plus they're far cheaper than gym membership!

The key to whipping your body into shape is to make sure you build up to a variety of different forms of exercise each week. That way you're less likely to get bored, plus you'll tone up different parts of your body. So try swimming (burns almost 200 calories in half an hour), then power-walking (300 calories in half an hour), plus have an exercise-video session or do a few sets of press-ups – great for toning your bust. Yoga is a great way to firm up your flabby bits and wipe the stress from your face. In fact, one study found that Hatha yoga reduces stress levels even more than having a rest!

How did
it go?

Q I'm not a gym person and the thought of weightlifting or aerobics is a turn-off. Any suggestions?

A   *Do something you enjoy. Book a skiing holiday (skiing can burn as many as 600 calories per hour) or sign up for salsa lessons. Dancing is a great cardio exercise because it raises the heart rate and lowers stress levels and blood pressure, plus you can burn 250 to 500 calories in one hour. Also, when you do an activity you enjoy, the body releases serotonin, a 'happy' hormone that also lowers blood pressure.*

Q Is exercising indoors or outdoors most effective?

A   *One Australian study showed that the natural endorphin high you get from exercise is greater when you exercise outdoors. Moreover, exercising outdoors means you get a good boost of vitamin D from sunlight, which is good for bones, teeth and cell growth. Just five to ten minutes a day can help relieve symptoms of SAD (seasonal affective disorder), such as sleep problems, fatigue, anxiety and irritability. Exercising outside can also leave you sunkissed, but make sure you always wear sunscreen.*

Q What if I don't have the time to fit exercise into my life?

A   *Don't worry. A study found that three ten-minute sessions of exercise produce the same beneficial results as one thirty-minute session and can be easier to fit into your day. Besides, harder exercise doesn't necessarily bring greater psychological benefits, as just ten or twenty minutes of exercise can release chemicals that improve your mood.*

25

Can beauty products help you slim?

Lotions, potions and treatments promise all kinds of miracles, including inch loss and wobble firming. But are they worth the money?

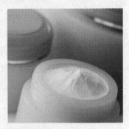

It's an appealing idea. Rub in this cream twice a day for six weeks and your flab will melt away.

A friend of mine once remarked that these creams should come with a symbol on them, featuring a slice of cake with a cross through it meaning that to lose weight, you have to watch what you eat as well as, or even rather than, spend money on some gimmicky product. But he's a cynic and a man – and men generally don't believe in the powers of applying creams to themselves. They prefer it if you do it for them, coupled with a back rub, after eating a fabulous meal you've cooked for them, and that you've also shopped for and cleaned up after – not to mention put the kids to bed, fed the cat and done a little recreational vacuuming. But enough man-bashing. This idea is as much for them as it is for women.

Depending on your background, beauty treatments can be very useful for getting in shape or a waste of time, money and effort. The cosmetics industry is always able to wheel out a boffin from their laboratories to produce clinical studies proving that X

Here's an
idea for
you...

Get a fake tan. It can make you look slimmer and leaner by sculpting, shadowing and highlighting muscles and curves. For the best results, have it applied in a salon. It will usually last for about five days.

cream really does help you lose inches, refine your silhouette or firm your curves. Meanwhile, most other doctors and scientists will say that what you apply from the outside doesn't make a blind bit of difference. Advertising claims are strictly regulated and can only go so far, so it can be hard to know how effective these products really are. The better magazines and newspapers do some investigatory work and produce information and recommendations of their own.

I believe that some of these treatments do have an effect, though it might be short-lived. I also think that the psychological element can't be underestimated. There's no doubt that looking after yourself does make you feel good. When you feel good, you're motivated, positive and confident, which is how you need to feel to spur you on to losing weight.

Here are my opinions of what's on offer:

SALON TREATMENTS

These usually involve being wrapped, massaged or painlessly zapped with some sort of electrical current. Massage is undoubtedly soothing and is claimed to stimulate your lymphatic system, which drains waste fluid from your tissues. You'll feel good afterwards, but not thinner. Wraps can shrink inches, but it's just fluid loss – they are fab for feeling a bit thinner for a special occasion. You can't beat them for a short-term boost. Electrical impulses stimulate your muscles by working them while you lie back and read a magazine. You would see better results with regular exercise.

'After forty a woman has to choose between losing her figure or her face. My advice is to keep your face and stay sitting down.'
BARBARA CARTLAND

Defining idea...

FAT-BUSTING CREAMS

Despite the claims, I really don't believe you get results unless you eat less and move more too. Still, they do make your skin feel very smooth and soft and strokable.

COLONIC IRRIGATION

This is very controversial. It is based on the principle that toxic deposits are stored in your large intestine. When these are flushed out, it kickstarts the metabolism and helps elimination. If having a speculum inserted in your anus and having gallons of water sloshing around your insides is your idea of a good time, go right ahead! While many alternative practitioners say it's perfectly safe and even emotionally rewarding, conventional doctors reject the idea, even saying it's downright dangerous.

How did it go?

Q **A friend recommended skin brushing as a way to combat cellulite. Will it work?**

A *I am a fan of skin brushing. This is where you stroke a dry bristle brush in sweeping movements over your limbs and torso, always working towards the heart. It definitely makes your skin feel great and gets the circulation going. I don't think it will get rid of cellulite, though used in combination with massage, diet and exercise, it will help to hold it at bay.*

Q **I read about some slimming tights recently. Can you tell me more?**

A *Coffee tights look like normal tights but are impregnated with caffeine which slowly gets absorbed through the skin. The idea is that this speeds up the metabolism, leading to inch loss. One test had all the volunteers losing inches from their waists and hips. Usually I'd be cynical, but I think I might just give these a go myself. You can find out more at www.palmers-shop.com.*

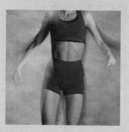 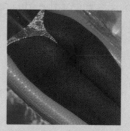

26

The blushing bride

But are the blushes for the right reasons? Yes, you've dreamed about this day since you were a little girl, but remember you had the figure of a twelve year old back then. It's a must to be realistic when searching for the right dress.

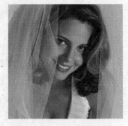

Always wanted to shimmer in silk but know going bra free is out of the question? Tried on a full skirt and looked like the Christmas fairy (tree included)? The trick is to choose a dress that you like, but a dress that suits you as well.

Firstly, you must not go into a bridal shop with any fixed ideas; that way madness lies. All kinds of married women will tell you that the dress they tried on for a laugh, the dress they would never have considered in a million years, turned out to be the one they tripped up the aisle in. So leave trawling the wedding magazines until you have had at least one major trying-on session.

Here's an idea for you...

When choosing your dress, think first about your hairstyle and headdress, or absence of one. Different necklines will work better with hair up or down, with veil or without, so consider these ideas. Tiaras are a popular choice and suit any length of hair, although you may need styling products and pins to help them stay put. If you want a headdress with a minimum of fuss, a simple silk Alice band or headband can be cute and 50s retro while also allowing for a windy day (Highland weddings take note). Coronets look wonderful with a long veil, and fresh flowers bring simple charm to any dress; a single exotic bloom can add real glamour. Hats need a more formal outfit, but can look dynamite with a chic trouser or skirt suit. Just bear in mind you might want to take it off later, and you'll need a hairdo that can handle it.

Your wedding dress is unlike any dress you will ever have worn. For starters, it is likely to be white or cream, and much longer, and a much more unusual shape, than anything currently hanging in your wardrobe. So throw away your preconceptions of what will suit you: you'll be wrong. Try on every shape you can get your hands on, even if you don't like the style. You are guaranteed to be surprised by what flatters you. And that goes for your complexion, too: pure white doesn't work for everyone so make sure you see the dress against your skin in daylight as well as in the shop, because your guests will.

When you have found a style that suits, compare the cost of materials. (A plain silk shift is likely to differ from a boned, beaded bodice with full skirt.) This will give you an idea of what you need to consider when setting your budget. Now you can look at the wedding magazines, to help you find variations on your theme. Bear in mind, you will need to order at least three to four months before your big day and, if you are indecisive, work back from this date to make sure you don't end up panic buying.

ANYONE COVERING YOUR BACK?

You need a dress buddy to talk you out of any childish Cinderella fantasy and give her free rein to say, 'Yes, your bum does look big in that'. (When you say your vows, most guests won't be looking at your face.) And make sure one of you remembers to bring some heels, unless you will be wearing flat (or no) shoes. Having your dress cut a few inches too short could be devastating, sartorially speaking.

'*I...chose my wife, as she did her wedding gown, not for a fine glossy surface but such qualities as would wear well.*'
OLIVER GOLDSMITH, *The Vicar of Wakefield.*

Defining idea...

SOME NOT-SO-EXCITING PRACTICAL CONSIDERATIONS

A lace shift in December? Nice idea; miserable wedding. Think about the season of your wedding. In high summer, cool silk, chiffon, pure cotton or lace; cooler winter months call for heavier fabrics such as brocade, velvet and duchess satin. And be practical: hiking a huge skirt through fields to a marquee might seem funny at first but will soon lose its humorous appeal.

Be positive. Write a list of all your best assets and those which you would like to show off to full advantage on the day. (Not all of them will be suitable for showing off.) A lovely off-the-shoulder number is ideal for a high neck, and a pear shape can be hidden with a slinky waist, flaunting a full skirt and nipped-in bodice. You will never have a chance to hide your disliked bits so skilfully again! And don't forget that budgets often get stretched by essentials such as underwear, stockings, shoes, jewellery, bags, scarves, etc. All will add finishing touches and complete your look, but will they bust your budget?

109

How did it go?

Q **The wedding is off. I've found my dream dress and *he* says no, it's too expensive for a one-off. What can I do?**

A *Ah, men and frocks. There are ways of reining in the costs while letting your dreams run free; consider man-made fabrics instead of silk. If you want to feel the real McCoy of silk on your skin, consider hiring your dress. Before you shriek in horror, you can pay about the same to hire a designer dress as you would to buy a mass-produced one. If you must have it, you could recoup some of the cost of a designer dress by selling it after the wedding. Lots of agencies and web sites offer this service (unless you've covered it in red wine). And how often will you wear it anyway?*

Q **No, I can't bear to part with my dress. What should I do now?**

A *Then something might have to give. Offer to compromise on another area of the wedding and tell him the dress will be a family heirloom. Preserve your dress by having it expertly cleaned and boxed, ready for your offspring's big day. Or cut it short and dye it red, and take him dancing...*

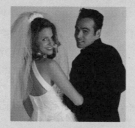 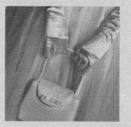 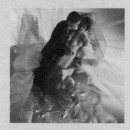

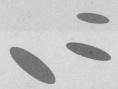

110

27

A good dressing down

Less is sometimes more but conversely when it comes to looking sexy, flesh is sometimes less. Learn the art of leaving something to the imagination.

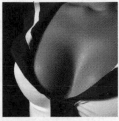

There's nothing as off-putting as someone who is trying too hard to look sexy. And the easiest way to do this is to dress 'too young' when we've left twenty-five far behind.

Sex appeal has a lot to do with confidence. My aunt, a very chic Italian lady, always told me as a gawky teenager to try to look a bit more frivolous. She would casually throw a shawl over my shoulders and tell me to 'carry it'. At the time I had no idea what she was talking about. Now I understand that she was trying to get me to wear clothes in a sexy manner, to ooze confidence and frivolity.

So how does one do it? The first thing is not to wear anything uncomfortable. It's very hard to look oh-so-cool if your bra-strap is digging into your ribs. Second, don't wear anything too risky. The skirt riding up to reveal a red g-string is not a classy look. I once wore one of those T-shirts with huge holes for the arms that were all the rage in the 80s. As I walked down the entire length of a double-decker bus to get off at Hyde Park Corner I noticed the whole, totally packed, bus staring at me. 'I

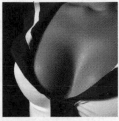

111

Here's an idea for you...

Go commando. Going out without wearing your underwear makes you feel amazingly sexy. And it's a secret only you know, until you decide to share it with your partner of course...

must be looking particularly hot today,' I thought to myself. It wasn't until I got off the bus that I noticed the T-shirt was half-way across my chest. And in those days I didn't wear a bra. Another equally devastating incident came when I went on my first date with a demi-god whom I had been lusting after for months. As I put my arms back to let the maître d' take my coat, both my hold-up stockings fell to my ankles. Great start. So safety first, wear stuff you know won't embarrass you.

You may be tempted to under-dress. And by that I mean wearing something so short it may as well not be there, thinking this looks sexy. Although men like a woman to be in touch with her inner tramp, most don't necessarily want the rest of the world to see their date looking like a lap dancer. The look you need to master is sexy but classy – chic and elegant with a hint of raunchy for the girls, and well turned out at all times for the guys. (Personally, I find pink shirts irresistible, but others may not.)

If your twenties have been and gone it is essential to avoid the mutton dressed as lamb look. If you are over forty, be proud of it. There is no reason why you can't be sexy, but think refined and subtle like Audrey Hepburn, and not Britney Spears.

This idea of having a model in your mind when you shop is a useful one. Before investing in those sequined trousers ask yourself whether your icon would wear them.

The way clothes feel to the touch is also important, especially if you're aiming for body contact, so think about wearing clothes that follow the contours of your body and that are made of sensual fabrics such as silk, cashmere, velvet, mohair, chiffon and chenille.

There is such a lot of choice out there and the way you dress will make a huge difference to how you feel, how you sit in a chair, how you walk down the street. Which in turn determines how sexy you'll be.

'Clothes maketh the man.'
Early fifteenth century proverb

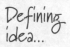

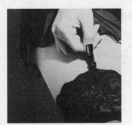

How did it go?

Q **I don't really know what looks good on me and make too many fashion errors. How can I avoid them?**

A *Go to a big department store and hire a professional shopper to advise you. This will cost a bit of money but you only need do it once and then you can take her advice with you on every shopping trip you ever make. You'll probably find that your shopper chooses things for you that you would never have gone for yourself. This can be very liberating and transform your view about what you can and should wear.*

Q **I am always unsure of the sort of image I will project. I have a hot date coming up and want to make a good first impression – can you help?**

A *There are a couple of basic rules. If you wear light colours you will come across as more innocent and vulnerable. If you wear bold colours you will seem in charge. Think about your date, what would appeal to him? If you want to look sexy but in a completely unobvious way, then wear clothes that if he were to undress you would guide him, for example a shirt with buttons down the front or a dress with a zip all the way down the back. Men find the thought of what is underneath the zip or buttons intriguing.*

28

Get bikini fit

**Looking beautiful when wearing very little requires
specialist tactics.**

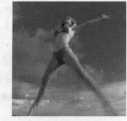

Also, there are rules to buying a bikini
that shouldn't be broken unless you're
under sixteen, Ursula Andress or model–slim with
buttocks you could crack nuts with.

First, take a long look at your body in a full-length mirror. Assess your proportions
and establish your body shape. Are you a pear, an apple, wonderfully hour-glass,
top-heavy, saddled with saddlebags or just plain, um, voluptuous? Decide which bits
you'd like to hide and which bits you'd like to display with pride.

Now take a look at the tips below. Think of them as your cut-out-and-keep guide to
bikini shopping. The truth is, you can still wear a bikini if you have a less than
model-like body. You just need some poolside savvy, such as what cuts, colours and
shapes to choose, i.e. what cups to go for to flaunt your good bits and how to cause
a distraction from the bad. (Screaming that there's someone drowning isn't the only
option!)

Here's an idea for you...

Before splashing out on that gorgeous new bikini, make sure it fits comfortably and is also practical in the changing room. Check that it does actually contain you and your curves when you're moving by running on the spot and raising your arms up and down. Also ensure the bottoms won't ride up uncomfortably by doing a few squats or kneeling down.

FLAT- OR SMALL-CHESTED?

The best techniques for boosting small busts include wearing padded bras and tops with frilly details or horizontal stripes. You could also try underwired bras with bows or flowers that'll add an extra dimension to an otherwise uneventful bustline.

PEAR-SHAPED OR BIG-BOTTOMED?

Think carefully about bikini bottoms. Try tie-sided briefs. They're really flattering on bigger hips. Also, you can adjust them to fit perfectly and the ties detract from any lumps and bumps. Alternatively, choose bikinis with boyish shorts or flippy skirts.

WHAT ABOUT COLOUR?

If you're trying to minimise a curvaceous bum and enhance a smaller bust, try a solid dark colour on the bottom and put the colour and pattern on top. Big boobs, small bum? Reverse the rules.

BUSTY?

There's nothing sexy about huge knockers if you own a pair of them and are trying to squeeze them into swimwear. So, in order to draw attention away from your boobs to your face and at the same time lengthen your torso, go for V-neck swimsuits or bikinis. These will draw the eye from your décolletage downwards, effectively carving your bust in two. Another good tip to minimise a hefty bust is to choose thick shoulder straps.

'There is no excellent beauty that hath not some strangeness in the proportion.'
SIR FRANCIS BACON

Defining idea...

BIG TUMMY?

Opt for vest tops with built-in support, which are great at covering a bulging tummy. Alternatively, go for high-cut bikini bottoms that come higher over your abdomen.

Once you hit the beach:

- Sit and take huge deep breaths of that lovely fresh sea air, which can calm your mind and spirit and also help you sleep better.
- Think of the beach as an outdoor gym. Don't just lounge, get swimming – one of the best all-over body exercises as it works every major muscle group. Also, it's low-impact so it puts no strain on your joints.
- Try wading through hip-height water. This is a great lower-body toner and can really help firm bottoms and thighs. And running across the sand barefoot is good for toning calf muscles, plus you can exfoliate your feet at the same time.
- If you're feeling very comfortable in your bikini, a game of beach volleyball can burn up to about 300 calories in just thirty minutes and targets bums, thighs, pecs and wobbly arms.

How did it go?

Q What's the best way to make my broad shoulders look more feminine?

A *Think about the neckline. A U-neck swimsuit or bikini top will make you look narrower and slighter.*

Q I look huge in my gorgeous new patterned bikini yet I followed all your rules. What went wrong?

A *How big is the pattern? If you went for a large motif, chances are it's making you look fleshier than you are. The best rule in terms of patterns is to make sure the motif is smaller than your fist. That way it won't beef up your bits.*

Q You mentioned Ursula Andress and I love those belted bottoms she wore in *Dr No*. Do they suit everyone?

A *The great news is that yes, they do. As well as being sexy, they're rather ingenious because the belt actually helps create a waist, which makes women look instantly slimmer round the middle. Who knows, Ursula Andress may well have been trying to disguise her own wobbly bits.*

29

Want to know a secret?

Cellulite is fat – there's no getting round this. So drop some pounds and you'll shift some cellulite. Try these weight loss tips.

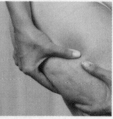

Oh, if we had a penny for every column inch devoted to that mischievous demon cellulite, we'd be zillionaires. Orange-peely dimples are not some mysterious skin condition or bizarre freak of biology. Experts around the globe are pretty unanimous about one thing: cellulite is fat. Simple as that.

More specifically it's actually the top layer of fat, just beneath your skin, known as subcutaneous fat. When scientists conducted tests on the dimpled skin we get on our bottoms, tummy and thighs, they discovered that it was exactly the same kind of fat as that found on the rest of our body.

However, there's a reason why it looks different than the skin on the rest of your body. It comes down to the tissue that connects the fat to your skin and keeps it in

Here's an idea for you...

Want quick results? Try brushing shimmery bronzer on the backs of legs or thighs or smother thighs with a light-reflecting cream or lotion. They catch the light, making legs look smoother, and draw attention away from your cellulitey bits.

place. This tissue is made from collagen fibres known as septae, which, in women, run in a kind of criss-cross fashion like honeycomb.

So far, so straightforward.

But when a woman gains weight, the fat cells swell, and the fat effectively bulges out between the fibres. Imagine what sausage looks like as it bursts out of its skin, or how stuffing can bulge out of an old mattress and you get an idea of what happens in your thighs and bottom. When the fat bulges out between the fibres, the result is those domed-shaped dimples we know as cellulite.

The reason why we get it on our bottoms and thighs is because when women gain weight, Mother Nature ensures the extra fat goes on our thighs, bum and tum as all those pear-shaped women out there will testify. What's more, even women who are slim elsewhere can be afflicted by cellulite, thanks to the distribution of fat.

Fortunately, getting down to your ideal weight through diet and exercise means you'll shed the fat that causes cellulite.

Start by taking a long hard look at yourself. Could you shed a few pounds? Chances are, the answer is yes. Nearly half of us are overweight. Your medical practitioner, your gym instructor or a (brutally honest) friend can also help assess your weight.

Or try working out your body mass index (BMI). Your BMI is basically your weight in kilograms divided by your height in metres squared. So if you are 10 stone 4 lb (65 kg) and 5 ft 4 in (1.62 m), your BMI is just under 25: $65 \div (1.62 \times 1.62) = 24.8$

You can check out your BMI according to the following ranges, as used by the World Health Organisation:

Less than 18.5	underweight
18.5–24.9	healthy weight
25–29.9	overweight
30–34.9	obese
35–39.9	very obese
40 or more	extremely obese

If your BMI is more than 25, it's time to shift some fat.

Start small. Make some changes to your diet, such as cutting down on your fat intake, and swap processed, refined carbs – such as white bread and cakes – for wholegrains. Start taking gentle exercise: aim for 30 minutes of aerobic exercise at least three times a week. Brisk walking is a good place to start.

'You are drunk Sir Winston, you are disgustingly drunk.' 'Yes Mrs Braddock, I am drunk. But you, Mrs Braddock are ugly and disgustingly fat. And in the morning, I will be sober.'
SIR WINSTON CHURCHILL

Defining idea...

Try these five golden rules today to kickstart your weight loss:

■ Eat breakfast – as long as it's not a fatty fry up. Experts have found that dieters who eat a high-fibre breakfast lose more weight than dieters who skip breakfast.

■ Make sure you get your five portions of fruit and veg a day. Make them a priority before you eat anything else – you'll feel fuller already and will get more nutrients into your diet.

■ Never say never to treats. Depriving yourself of your favourite foods often makes you want to rebel – and you can end up bingeing. Instead, just have a tiny amount and use a teaspoon instead of a dessert spoon. Learn to savour instead of scoff.

■ Eat snacks. Yes, honestly! Eating healthy snacks – fruit, pitta breads and hummous, nuts and yoghurt helps keep your blood sugar levels steady – you'll never get hungry, so will be less likely to reach for cakes and chocolate. Aim to eat a low-fat snack every two hours.

■ Watch your portions: some people swear they eat healthily yet never lose weight. Huge portions may be the problem. You should be aiming for no more than a fistful of carbs and protein at one meal. But fill up with plenty of veggies.

Q   Why don't men get cellulite?

A   *Because it's a man's world, that's why. And because men's skin is thicker so their subcutaneous fat is less noticeable. Also, men's connective fibres, which hold the fat in place, are different – theirs run diagonally, so effectively hold the fat down better. Plus they're less prone to getting fat than us, thanks to the male hormone testosterone, and when they do it's around the tum rather than the bottom and thighs.*

Q   So cellulite is a hormone thing is it?

A   *Kind of. Female hormones are responsible for the distribution of fat over our bottom, thighs and tummy. Oestrogen also encourages fluid retention, which causes women's fat cells to bulge out more. Some women find that their cellulite gets worse when they're taking the contraceptive pill, or during or after pregnancy because their hormone levels surge. The more body fat you have, the more oestrogen you produce, so it's a vicious circle. But watching your weight can help.*

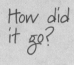
How did it go?

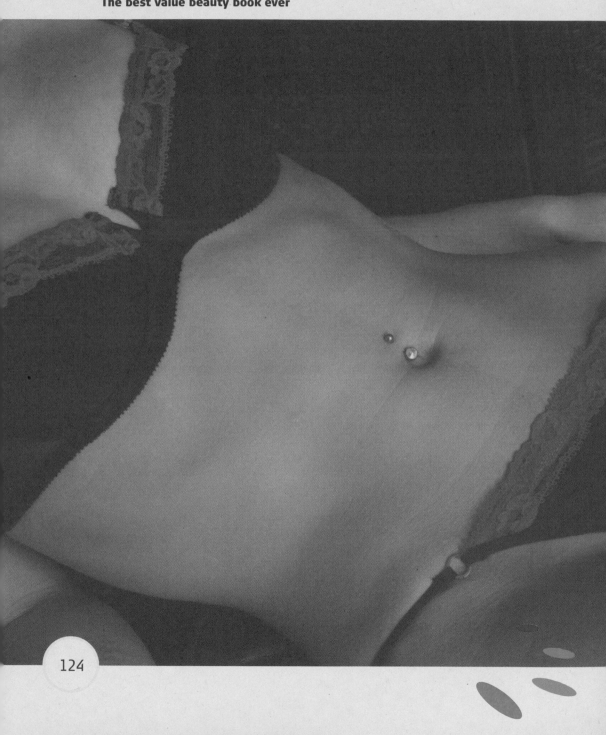

30

The power of lovely lingerie

Underwear. It's crucial. Get it right and you feel great. It's an essential part of being incredibly sexy.

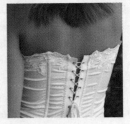

It boosts your confidence and helps you look marvellous in and out of your clothes. What's not to love?

When I first travelled to the continent I was amazed at all the little underwear shops selling smalls at what I thought were extortionate prices. I reasoned that there was nothing wrong with a pack of five knickers for the price of one bra-strap in some chichi shop. Up to a point I was right. There are days when those cotton no-frills knickers work well. But what is truly different about your average French-woman, is that she will wear sexy matching bra and knickers every day. And she is prepared to spend around £60 on each ensemble.

Now that I live in France I have gone very French in my attitude towards underwear. My bra and knicker drawers are stuffed full of matching ensembles. And oddly enough, once I started on this gig, I found it hard to go back to the five-packs. There's something empowering about matching top and bottom and for this reason you should seriously consider buying at least two pairs of knickers with each bra. To

Here's an idea for you...

This expensive underwear is all very well, but a pain to hand wash. I take mine into the shower with me and wash it there, which is much easier. It also means you don't end up with that awful grey shade of white as your smalls get washed on a 60 degree cycle with all the wrong colours. Treat it well, and it will last much longer.

make sure you don't suffer from the dreaded VPL under trousers always make at least one of these pairs a g-string, or try out French knickers or boxer shorts for girls – no VPL and damn sexy!

Sex appeal has a lot to do with confidence and there is nothing like good underwear to enhance your body shape and make you feel more attractive. For the flatter-chested among us, there is no more comforting moment than pulling a T-shirt over a new Wonderbra and seeing our body shapes totally transformed. For larger ladies, a good well-fitting bra is even more essential. If you want to minimise your bust under business suits, get measured by an expert to find out your correct cup size – you will lose 10 lbs, I swear, immediately you put on the right fitting bra. And if you want to emphasise your cleavage, a right fitting bra does this stupendously well, besides being much more comfortable.

A sexy g-string can work wonders for your buttocks. Some people find them incredibly uncomfortable – I did to begin with – but once you get used to them you will hardly ever wear ordinary knickers again.

If you're wearing the right underwear, you feel like you can take on the world. It makes you feel so much more confident. You walk into a business meeting and although the others can't see what you've got on underneath your suit, you know, and it gives you a sense of superiority. I spoke to Chantal Thomass, France's leading underwear designer, on this subject. 'Lingerie is fundamental to the way a woman feels,' she says. 'If your underwear isn't right, nothing else works.' A friend of mine says it determines her whole mood for the day: 'It's the first thing I put on and it puts me in a good or bad mood,' she says. 'I have a very intimate relationship with my lingerie, after all it is the thing I put on next to my skin.'

'A lady is one who never shows her underwear unintentionally.'
LILLIAN DAY, American author

Defining idea...

As we all know, for whatever reason, men *adore* stockings and suspenders. Just about every man I know is totally gone on them. 'I don't know what it is about them,' says one. 'They just drive me wild. Maybe it's because all the Playboy models I lusted over in my youth wore them.' Our job here is not to analyse, just wear them. Classic black suspender belts are the best but red can be good for a special occasion, adding an extra sex-vixen allure. The great thing about kinky or sexy underwear is that it enhances your sex drive as well as your partner's. You're hardly going to sit around feeling like a drudge in a pair of red crotchless knickers!

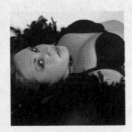

How did it go?

Q I don't really have the confidence to go dressing up in strange underwear. What do you suggest?

A *Who said anything about it having to be strange? You could start with a very classic matching bra and knickers. Even if you can't afford La Perla, you should check it out and see if you can source a cheaper version somewhere. It is the most stunning underwear ever and will give you an idea of how crucial underwear can be. If you're wearing a La Perla all-in-one the sky's the limit...Wolford isn't bad either and much cheaper, although still not a steal. Check out the sales – most large department stores stock Wolford. They do brilliant tights and stockings as well, so are well worth looking at. If you look after them (i.e. don't ladder them or put them in the washing machine) they can last for several years. Check them out at www.wolford.com*

Q How about sexy underwear for us blokes?

A *Now you're talking. Amazingly, men are catching up. There are some great websites now offering all sorts of goodies, including the very slinky l'homme invisible. Totally irresistible. There's also a solution for men who feel nature has been a little stingy in the lunch-box department. A website (go find it if you're really interested) is offering two models of padded pants: colt or stallion (oh please). The blurb promises the padding is discreetly tucked away in hidden pockets and will change your life. Until you take your knickers off, that is.*

31

Great gnashers

**Confidence, good looks and success are the kind of qualities
a brilliant smile can impart. Dig out that floss today.**

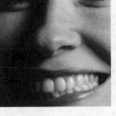

I've always been a bit obsessed with
teeth, as I had braces as a child. A full
Hannibal Lecter number that tortured my poor
wayward teeth into meek submission and earned
me odd stares on the school bus.

As a result, I notice every detail about someone's smile – veneers, caps, chips,
crowns, the works. I assess the teeth of everyone I meet with my own kind of
Playtex barometer: 'has she or hasn't she?' When British starlets go off to Hollywood
in search of stardom and come back with newly bleached, chiselled, perfected teeth
it's as obvious to me as if they'd come back with a third breast.

Being a teeth person, I look at people with a naturally beautiful smile with awe. It's
the first thing I notice about someone. Imperfect teeth can make the seemingly
beautiful less so. And a gorgeous set of pearlies can transform the merely plain into
a radiant beauty. Psychologists say this is quite a normal reaction. Apparently, we
assign negative character traits to people with a bad dental appearance.

Here's an idea for you... **Stained teeth? Try this old wives' tale: add a drop of clove oil to your toothpaste before brushing your teeth to help brighten your smile.**

Having a pleasant smile makes you appear not just more attractive, but also more honest and trustworthy. And when you smile a beautiful smile, you make the person you're smiling at feel better and generate warmth, happiness and confidence.

Your teeth can even make you look younger. Anthropologists say that this is because white and even teeth, healthy pink gums and a convex smile are characteristics of youth. However, as the years go by, our teeth lose their luminosity and become dull, stained and chipped. A mouthful of fillings can also make your smile look dull and grinding your teeth can wear them down. So, taking care of them and investing in the odd procedure (whitening, straightening, etc.) can actually take years off you.

Considering all these plus points, it's little wonder that we're spending a fortune on our teeth these days and that there's a cosmetic dentist on every high street. To keep your teeth looking their best try the following:

- Dentists say it's vital to use a meticulous cleaning routine and to use the best tooth products you can. Brush your teeth at least twice a day and ideally after each meal.
- Make sure you visit your dentist regularly – at least every twelve months – and never miss a check up.
- If needs be, invest in cosmetic procedures or braces. Amazing techniques are available these days and full-on braces are a thing of the past.

- Floss at least once a day.
- Cut down on sugary snacks and try fruit, vegetables and calcium-rich low-fat yoghurt instead. If you must eat something sweet stick to chocolate, as with chewy sweets the sugar gets sloshed around in your mouth for longer.
- Finish meals with cheese, which helps neutralise the acid in your mouth and therefore helps prevent tooth decay. Cheese is rich in calcium and phosphorous and this helps replace some of the minerals in tooth enamel, thereby strengthening teeth.
- Chew gum. Look for brands that contain xylitol because it's been found to help protect against – even reverse – tooth decay. Xylitol is found naturally in berries, mushrooms, lettuce and corn on the cob, too.
- Avoid stain-causing culprits such as coffee, tea, cigarettes and red wine. Try a whitening toothpaste to brighten your smile and have your teeth cleaned by a hygienist every six months.

Are you brushing correctly? And for long enough? In order to clean all your tooth surfaces thoroughly you need to spend at least two minutes at it each time. The brushing motion itself helps remove stains, so don't cheat!

'A smile is an inexpensive way to change your looks.'
CHARLES GORDY, author

Defining idea…

- First, focus on the inner and outer surfaces of your teeth. Place your toothbrush at a 45-degree angle and use gentle, short, tooth-wide strokes following your gum line. To clean the inside surfaces of front teeth, tilt your brush vertically and use gentle up-and-down strokes with the toe of your brush.
- Then move on to your chewing surfaces, holding your brush flat and brushing back and forth.
- Next, brush your tongue. Use a back-to-front sweeping method to remove food particles, which will also help freshen your mouth.
- Finally, gently brush the roof of the mouth.

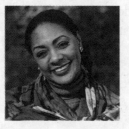 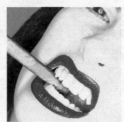 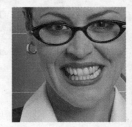

Q   **What can I do to stop grinding my teeth at night?**

A   *Grinding your teeth may be a sign of stress or a less than perfect bite. It's often responsible for aching jaws and neck pain, and can damage your teeth as it often causes cracks that can attract stains. See your dentist who will check your bite and make you a preventive gumshield to wear while you're sleeping.*

Q   **I suspect I have bad breath. What can I do?**

A   *Bad breath often comes down to poor dental hygiene, as the smell is the result of bacteria breaking down those bits of food that are left in your mouth. Visit your dentist, as tooth decay can cause bad breath. And make sure you brush your teeth and tongue at least twice a day. Floss, too, to get rid of plaque. Try to finish off meals with fruit and always aim to drink plenty of water because dehydration reduces saliva flow, which can make the problem worse. Breath mints and fresheners are good, but they only work temporarily. Always eat breakfast to stimulate the flow of saliva, which helps get rid of morning breath.*

Q   **What is the best way to whiten my teeth?**

A   *You can get some great whitening toothpastes these days that produce fantastic results. Alternatively, try laser-assisted bleaching, which is available on most high streets and only takes about an hour. Or investigate tray bleaching, where you wear a tray containing bleaching solution for a short period each day for a week or longer. Another option is ultra-thin veneers, which are bonded to your teeth and can make your teeth straighter as well as whiter.*

How did it go?

133

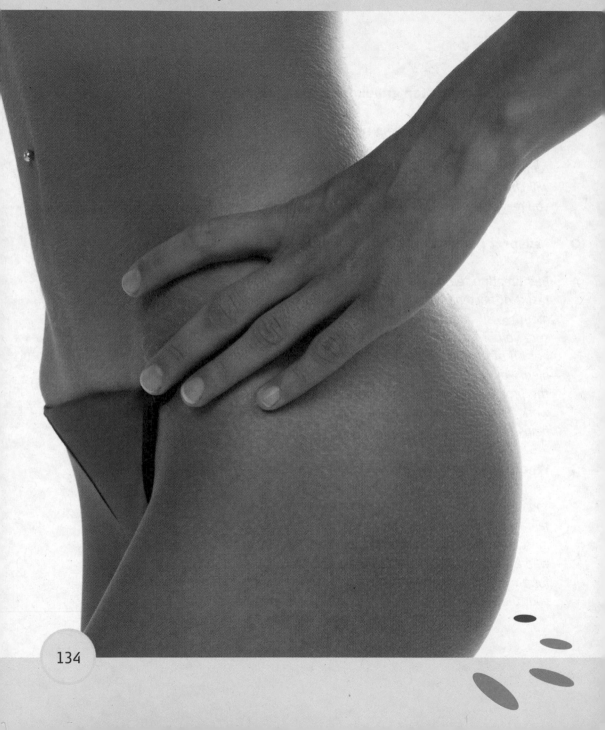

32

Give it the brush-off

Here's a cheap and cheerful solution to your cellulite woes. Daily skin brushing can help soften and smooth out orange-peel thighs. And you'll soon see the results.

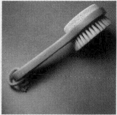

You'd be forgiven for thinking that you need a vast budget, and a coterie of beauty therapists and personal trainers to really banish cellulite.

But judging by some of those paparazzi shots of celebrities and glamourpusses baring cellulite-stricken thighs, having lots of cash clearly doesn't guarantee you a svelte, smooth behind. In fact one of the most inexpensive ways to tackle a dimply bottom is to give it a good firm brushing.

Most beauty experts and authorities on cellulite agree that regular body brushing can dramatically enhance the texture of your skin and help the dimples appear less noticeable.

The advantages are you can do it every day in the comfort and privacy of your own home, that it takes no more than three to five minutes of your time, and that it costs nothing – well, the cost of a bottle of wine for a decent brush. And that you can usually see results within days.

Here's an idea for you...

Get the circulation in your bottom and thighs going, and smooth the skin at the same time, with a home-made scrub. Mix two tablespoons of finely ground oatmeal together with one tablespoon of almond oil. Rub into the skin, then rinse off in the shower.

Body brushing can help minimise cellulite in two ways. Firstly, it helps remove surface dead cells, which makes the skin on your rear end look smoother and more even-textured. Think about how much smoother and more radiant your face looks after you've exfoliated; you get the same effect on your bum too!

Secondly, dry skin brushing is considered an effective way to stimulate circulation and boost lymphatic drainage – both of these systems are believed to be major contributing factors to cellulite.

Think about how blotchy and pasty your face looks when you've been sedentary or lolling about lazily for days on end in a centrally heated or air-conditioned room. Compare this to how it looks when you've taken some exercise, washed, exfoliated and patted your skin. Boosting your circulation improves skin dramatically.

In fact many experts describe cellulite as a disorder of the lymphatic drainage system and your circulation. When these two body systems work optimally, your circulation delivers oxygen and important nutrients to your cells via blood, and the lymphatic drainage system removes the waste-products.

Think, then, of the healthy fatty tissues on your bottom and thighs. This tissue has a blood supply which provides nutrients and oxygen, and a drainage system taking waste-products away. So far so good.

When this flow of fluid slows down, either because you live the life of a couch potato, or have a very sedentary job, your limbs don't get much action and your skin in that region suffers.

Think of your skin cells that separate the fat cells in your bottom and thighs as bits of elastic. The more sedentary you are, the less nourished they become, and gradually they become thicker and less elastic. If you're a confirmed couch potato, the continued sluggish movement of fluid round your body makes these fibres even thicker and tougher.

And, because these fibres lose their elasticity, the fat that lies beneath them ends up bulging out between them, creating the dimples we know as cellulite.

All of this is made even worse by the excess fluid in the bottom and thigh area – which is another result of poor lymph flow and circulation.

Dry skin brushing, then, can help get your circulation and lymph flowing again. Plus some experts also believe that skin brushing helps encourage new skin cells to regenerate and boost collagen production, which in turn helps elasticity.

Convinced? Judge for yourself. Try it every day before your shower or bath and brush your skin in long strokes towards the heart.

'The buttocks are the most aesthetically pleasing part of the body because they are non-functional...as near as the human form can ever come to abstract art.'
KENNETH TYNAN, legendary theatre critic (but clearly lacking even a basic knowledge of anatomy)

Defining idea...

HOW TO BODY-BRUSH

Start at your feet and brush your soles, toes and ankles and top of each foot gently but firmly with long, sweeping movements. Brush the front and back of your lower legs, working towards your knees. Then rest your foot against the bath or a chair and brush from your knees to your upper legs and thighs, waist and buttocks using long, smooth strokes. Repeat on both legs.

Many women get cellulite on their upper arms, so don't neglect your upper body. Start at your wrist and brush your inner arm in upward strokes towards your elbow. Then brush the palm of your hand, then the outer side of your hand, and move up towards the back of your arm. Repeat on the other arm. Follow with gentle circular movements over your stomach and chest.

Then shower or jump in the bath to remove the dead surface cells.

Q   Will a loofah do the trick for a skin brush?

A   *Yes, choose either a loofah or a body brush with natural fibres – they're gentler than man-made fibres. Aim to do it everyday before your shower or bath. The morning is a good time because it's invigorating and gets you revved up for your day. Then have a bath or shower to remove the dead skin cells. Wash your brush every few weeks with shampoo or warm water and leave it to dry.*

Q   Can I brush my skin when it's wet?

A   *You won't remove the surface cells so effectively if your brush is wet, neither will your brush glide so easily across your skin. The key is to use long, smooth movements towards the heart. Oh, and if you have a cellulitey tummy, brush that too, using very gentle circular movements – in a clockwise direction. Use very light pressure as this is a sensitive area.*

How did it go?

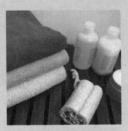
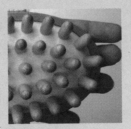

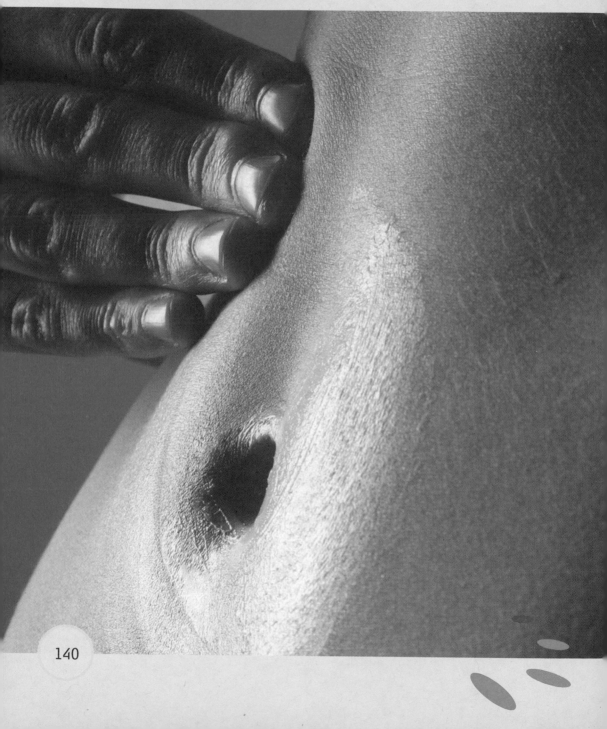

33

Beauty A–Z

When it comes to inner and outer beauty, there's more than one way to skin a cat.

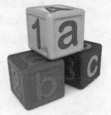

From the Alexander Technique to a zest for life, try these twenty-six beauty shortcuts to a more gorgeous, glamorous, confident and glowing you.

A: Alexander Technique
Good for improving your posture and relieving stress, muscle pain and injuries. Can even help you breathe better, too.

B: Balm
One little pot can go a long way. Rub it on your lips, use it to tame eyebrows and smooth cuticles, and dab it over make-up to give your cheeks a soft glow.

C: Vitamin C
Boosts immunity, is good for your heart, helps mop up free radicals and may protect you against cancer. Also great for skin and teeth, bones and gums. Best sources are blackcurrants, red peppers, oranges and kiwi fruit.

Here's an idea for you...

When exfoliating your face, smother the product over your hands too to whisk off any dead skin cells and make them look softer, smoother and younger.

D: Dandelion tea

A great diuretic that can help relieve bloating. It's also full of B vitamins. Swap your PG tips for a cup.

E: Eyebags

Leave a couple of teaspoons in the fridge, put them over your eyes as you lie down for ten minutes and you've got a cheap and cheerful fix.

F: Fringes

They can make your eyes look bigger, enhance your features and take years off you.

G: Gels

Anti-ageing gels and serums are better for oily skin than creams. Avoid overloading skin with moisturising creams that can make it oilier and prone to breakouts.

H: Humidifiers

A great way to keep skin hydrated if you're stuck in air-conditioned or central-heated rooms. Alternatively, put a bowl of water by a radiator at night to stop your skin drying out.

I: Indian head massage

Age-old therapy based on Ayurveda. Reviving, relaxing and rejuvenating.

J: Juniper oil
Stimulating and energising. Run yourself a bath and add a few drops now. Great for cellulite and as a skin tonic.

K: Kumquats
Yummy citrus fruit, rich in skin-friendly phytonutrients and bursting with vitamin C.

L: Leg-lengthening and Lunges
Lengthen your legs with a pair of floaty palazzo pants. They skim over all the bumps and draw the eye down. 'L' is also for lunges, which can tone up legs fast.

M: Mackerel
Full of essential fatty acids (EFAs) which are good for your skin, eyes, brain and mood. Aim to eat three portions of oily fish a week. Sardines, trout and fresh tuna are great sources of EFAs, too.

N: Nails
Nail nightmares? File them perpendicular to your finger and square them off; it's the best way to keep them chip free.

O: Optimism
Can boost your immune system, say scientists. How to get more of it? List ten good things that happened to you today.

P: Percale count
The weave measurement on linen. The higher the count, the softer and better it is for your skin. Good sheets help regulate body temperature, which aids sleep.

'Make the most of yourself,
for that is all there is of you.'
RALPH WALDO EMERSON

Q: Quickie stain remover

To remove stains on nails, dip them in lemon juice and then rub in some Vaseline to moisturise them.

R: Reiki

Japanese for 'universal life force'. It works on the premise that if your body's flow of energy stagnates, you're more prone to illness and low moods. It's a gentle touch massage; the practitioner lays her hands on you and you feel a lovely warm 'healing' heat move through your body.

S: Straight hair

Chic and looks great on a round face, as it can soften and narrow it. To make it ultra-sleek, blow-dry starting with the hair underneath and direct the nozzle to direct heat along the length of the hair. When it's dry, smooth down with ceramic straightening irons and add a mist of glossing spray.

T: Tan

Nothing slims, tones and lengthens like bronzed skin. The best fake tan? St Tropez is the choice of beauty gurus.

U: UVA and UVB rays

UVAs damage your skin's protective tissue and the cells that produce collagen, which keeps our skin elastic and line-free. Repeated damage to these cells can lead to skin cancer.

UVBs literally burn skin tissue and cause the redness and pain you associate with sunburn. Make sure you wear sunscreen at all times; nothing less than 15 SPF. Reapply regularly and use hair products with SPF protection to protect your hair too.

'Zest is the secret of all beauty. There is no beauty that is attractive without zest.'
CHRISTIAN DIOR

Defining idea...

V: Veins
Spider veins appear on the face and legs and worsen with age. Electrolysis, sclerotherapy or laser treatments are your options. Disguise them with concealer (applied after your foundation).

W: Writing
Studies show that keeping a diary or writing about your woes and worries can be an effective stressbuster and can help reduce fatigue.

X: X chromosomes
You got 'em, so flaunt 'em. Do something girly every day; try a face pack, buy some flowers, wear heels, go for cocktails with the girls. Treat yourself.

Y: Yoga
Your route to long, lean limbs and a balanced mind. If you like to sweat when you exercise, try Astanga, a dynamic cardio workout.

Z: Zest
Get more lemon in your life. It's a sunny cheerful colour, uplifting and warm. Lemons are tangy and full of the immune-boosting vitamin C, so try your own home-made lemonade.

How did
it go?

Q While we're on the A–Z theme, can I have another 'P' please, Bob?

A P is also for pores. They're the opening of a follicle with sebaceous glands and are usually more noticeable around the T-zone. They're also worse if your skin's oily and sadly get bigger as you get older because your skin loses its elasticity. There's nothing you can do to shrink them, but splashing cold water on your face can temporarily tighten them. Exfoliate regularly to keep them free of dead skin cells, try putting your make-up on in a downwards motion and avoid over-moisturising the area.

Q And another?

A 'P' is also for pictures of beautiful women to inspire you. Not stick insect supermodels, but the beauties captured by the world's artists such as Rubens, Michelangelo, Titian and Renoir. Invest in some wonderful art books for the coffee table to remind you that the beauty of real women – with curves and curls – transcends time.

34

Yes, we have no pyjamas

It's cold outside. In fact, it's cold inside. All you really want to do is to get into your full-length flannel nightie and snuggle up in bed.

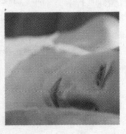

But you can't — not if you want to be sexy.

When asked what she wore in bed, Marilyn Monroe replied, 'Chanel No 5'. I'm not suggesting you wear nothing in the middle of winter but there are ways to avoid looking like a furry toy. The key is silk. There is nothing more comfortable and warm than a pair of silk pyjamas. OK, so there's probably not much that's more expensive either, but a good pair should last you for ever and you can go to bed knowing you look great and will be snug as a bug. While we're on the subject of splashing out on nightwear, a friend of mine once shocked the hell out of me by spending over £500 on a cashmere dressing gown from Ralph Lauren. I thought she'd gone totally bonkers. For £500 you could fly to the Caribbean. 'You could,' she said, 'but my dressing gown will be with me for ever.' Fifteen years later, she's still got it, and it looks great. Light, flowing, soft but oh so cosily warm. Total heaven. Working it out she's paid less than £40 a year to own this item – I now wish I'd bought one too.

Here's an idea for you...

When you are sleeping alone (not often, obviously, you sex-goddess), treat your hands and feet to a serious moisturising treatment. Put thick cream or oil on your feet and hands and massage well. This should be done once you're in bed so you don't kill yourself skidding over the floor to get there. Another good tip (strictly for when you're alone) is to put on a moisturising face pack and leave it on all night, and try to get to bed early. It's thought that an hour before midnight is worth two after.

Nightwear is a great thing to think about. It conjures up all sorts of sexy images. It is perhaps hard to believe but the sort of thing you wear at night can define your image. If you go to bed dressed like a Playboy bunny, chances are you'll get treated like one. Now that even high street stores sell sexy nightwear there is no longer any excuse for you to get into bed looking like a maiden aunt. It's all very well working hard all day long to look sexy, but it's essential to keep up that image at night-time too. This applies even if you are sleeping alone – it'll help reinforce your self-image as a sensual creature. Don't just give up and put on your grey (were once white) cotton jimjams. Think creatively, sexily and come up with something a little different. You can buy all sorts of cute little night outfits. Short nighties for example, simple cuts with perhaps a ribbon or two, even if they're made of cotton are a good choice. Please go for good quality though – polyester and other man-made fibres don't allow your skin to breathe, and while sweating is fine in bed, it should be from exertion not from simply overheating. Go for natural fibres such as cotton and silk, whatever design you choose. The one exception to this is when you're going for the Playboy look, in which case it needs to be red, glossy and totally fake – you probably won't end up keeping it on for long anyway.

'As you make your bed, so you must lie upon it.'
Late fifteenth century French proverb

Defining idea...

I like those little French knickers and tops ensembles. They can be very simple, and really cute – understatedly sexy, especially if they're made from cotton. They don't make you look like you're making a huge effort to look sexy, but are slightly different and popular with men who seem to find anything French irresistible.

You can also of course go for the Marilyn Monroe recipe and wear nothing but your favourite scent in bed. For this look you need to be smooth, soft and gorgeously clean or the effect will be lost. So wax, shave, whatever it is you do to stay stubble-free then shower or bath. An added bonus for soft skin is to exfoliate beforehand, preferably with exfoliating gloves. In fact if you do this three times a week you'll be amazed at the difference it makes. After exfoliating smother yourself with gorgeous smelling moisturising lotion or body oil. Similarly, don't overdo the scent, as there aren't many other smells in bed to detract from it. Try this trick; spray a cloud of it just in front of you and walk through it. You should come out the other end smelling just sweet enough.

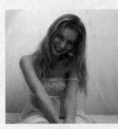

How did it go?

Q   Surely there's no point in all this? It's dark at night anyway?

A   *Wrong, of course there is a point. Your image is all-important, whatever the time of day or night. If you feel gorgeous you'll be more confident day and night. And anyway by the morning it will be light...*

Q   Some of this stuff is really expensive. Isn't it a waste to wear it at night?

A   *Don't think of it as just wearing it at night. We spend a quarter of our lives asleep, and probably more in bed. These hours take up a great chunk of your life and you need to be properly dressed. Obviously in order to be properly un-dressed.*

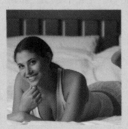
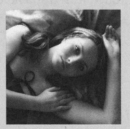

35

You look wonderful tonight

When you first met, you felt a little flutter every time you saw each other. Give your old flame first-date butterflies with a makeover that brings out the best in both of you.

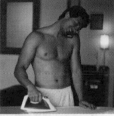

Just because he's seen your bikini line in 'relaxed' mode doesn't mean you can't still turn his head. All you need is a little application...

This idea won't make you look like a clown, or a celebrityholic style slave.

KEEP IT PERSONAL

Looking wonderful at short notice doesn't have to mean panic-buying clothes and products that sooner rather than later end up at the back of the wardrobe or bathroom cabinet. Many department stores offer a free personal shopper service for men and women. An hour's consultation is worth several trips rushing round the shops solo, and it's more likely to get you results. Be upfront. Explain that you want a look to make your long-term lover weak at the knees rather than weak at the stomach. The shopper should then bring you a selection of styles to suit your size, frame, personality and budget. The best ones won't force new trends on you, but adapt fashions to suit your style. It's up to you whether you love it or leave it.

Wouldn't it be great if you could take the afternoon off and spend it at a spa before meeting your partner in the evening? Most of us can't do this very often, but you can achieve a similar effect in about twenty minutes. Guys, pop into an old-fashioned barber's for a really close shave. Women, befriend a department store make-up counter assistant. Say something like, 'I'm happy with my look for work, but I want to look foxier in the evenings.' You'll get a free makeover, using all the latest tricks and techniques. 'Test' some new perfume as you go out and you're set to wow him.

Defining idea...

'You have to remember that before two hours of hair and make-up even I don't look like Cindy Crawford.'
CINDY CRAWFORD, modest supermodel

CUTTING EDGE

There's no quicker way to change your partner's reaction from ho-hum to wow than by blowing your budget at the hairdresser. A short back and sides, gamine crop or simply highlighting your tresses before having them professionally plaited and put up can transform you in your lunch hour. While we're talking about hair, be a smooth operator and get rid of any facial hair (nose and ears too).

HONEY I SHRUNK THE COSMETICS BILL

They say beauty is skin deep. But what do you do if you've run out of cleanser, toner or moisturiser, and you're going out in twenty minutes? Raid the cupboard. Honey will give you a gorgeous glow. It's a great cleanser and moisturiser combo, and smells delicious. Massage a little into your wet face and as you rub it off, it exfoliates all those dulling dead cells into the bargain. If you've got a little longer, mix a teaspoon of honey with a tablespoon of yoghurt and use it as a face mask. Or spread it on other rough, dry places, like feet, elbows or crispbread. Leave for ten minutes and rinse (or swallow). Take some in the shower with you too, as it's an ace conditioner that leaves your hair smelling delicious.

THE EYES HAVE IT

Get that come hither look by plucking your eyebrows into shape. Yes, even men – eyebrows that meet in the middle make you look like Dracula, and you know what trouble he had in keeping a woman! If you haven't got time to do full eye make-up, a whip of mascara can transform your look, drawing attention to your eyes. Many metrosexual men already know mascara also comes in clear.

HAND IT TO YOU

Eyes may be the windows of the soul, but when you reach out to touch your partner, how often is it with silky smooth hands rather than ones chapped and worn by washing up, gardening or typing? A callused caress isn't very sexy. If you usually work with your hands, it's time to get to work on your hands. Smooth rough hands by mixing some sea salt with some olive oil and rubbing it all over them. A few strokes with a nail buffer means you can leave nails in the buff, if you haven't time to polish up your act with varnish.

Defining idea…

'*As Ursula is my girlfriend of many years, I naturally rarely look at her anymore. I register that her outline is there, rather than actually looking at her. Purely for your benefit, however, I'll go rummaging around in the untidy basement of my memory to see if I can find where I left her features.*'
MIL MILLINGTON, newspaper columnist and author of *Things my Girlfriend and I Have Argued About*

153

How did it go?

Q My husband and I rub along pretty well, but it upsets me that he doesn't seem to appreciate the time and trouble I take to look good for him. I still have my figure, but he doesn't notice when I've had my hair done or bought a new frock. Is there anything I can do to knock him off his feet?

A *Sadly, some husbands just don't notice how their wives look and have little interest in their own appearance. It could be a sign of indifference, or that he's more interested in your inner beauty. Dress for yourself and enjoy the positive attention you get elsewhere.*

Q I'm not sure how to put this. I wish my girlfriend would make more of herself. She's a lovely person with little personal vanity, but she is up for new ideas. I'd like to get her a new outfit but don't know where to start. Any suggestions?

A *Lots of women's magazines use members of the public as models for before and after makeover features. The results can be dramatic. Nominate your girlfriend and give her a day she'll never forget. She'll learn lots of useful hints to help her make the most of her strong points and conceal the rest.*

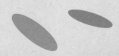

36

Creating curves

**A dainty waist means big sex appeal. Here's how to hone,
firm and whittle yours in weeks.**

Studies show that the waist to hip ratio —
going in and out in all the right places
— is a better gauge of a woman's attractiveness
than the size of her breasts.

The trouble is, these days we're so hung up on boobs. We know our bust size, our friends' bust size, our colleagues' bust size and the bust size of virtually every Hollywood actress and soap star on the box.

In our mother's day, waist size was the only statistic worth comparing. My mother always bangs on about the fact she got married with a 23-inch waist. Me, I'd have been pleased with a 23-inch thigh. But back then, waists were the measure of attractiveness; along with a squeaky clean reputation and a fetching ankle. By contrast, how many of us now even know the size of our waist?

We ought to because men of all cultures fancy women with small waists. Or to be precise, women with a 0.7 hip-to-waist ratio, i.e. waists that are 70% the size of their hips. And that doesn't necessarily involve being thin! Think Sophia Loren and

Here's an idea for you... **Invest in a gorgeous corset. Anything that boosts your bust and cinches your waist will do wonders for your rating in the bedroom.**

Marilyn Monroe. And although one recent study on *Playboy* centrefolds showed that women's waists are getting slightly wider, curves still reign supreme.

The reason for this is biological. A small waist that curves into a generous hip equals fertility and youth – it's a sign that a woman has high levels of oestrogen and low levels of testosterone. In fact, in studies of IVF patients, women with a hip to waist ratio of more than 0.8 were less likely to conceive. (Apparently having an index finger a couple of centimetres longer than your ring finger is another sign of high fertility.)

What's tricky about waists is that their size is largely inherited; you're either an apple shape, an hourglass or a pear. However, the good news is that you can trim an inch or so from your waist by losing weight and doing some waist-whittling exercises.

Love handles won't simply disappear. You have to shed the fat first. Experts say that if your waist measures between 81 and 89 cm (32–35 inches), you're overweight. If that's the case you'll need to follow a low-fat, low-cal diet and do three to five sessions a week of cardio exercise such as running, dancing, cycling or power walking.

WAIST-WHITTLING EXERCISES

'The curve is more powerful than the sword.'
MAE WEST

Defining idea...

Twist crunches
Lie on your back with your knees bent, your
feet flat on the floor and your fingers touching
your ears. Contract your abdominal muscles and slowly lift your torso off the floor.
When you can't lift any further, contract your side muscles and turn to the left.
Then return your torso to the floor and repeat on the other side. Build up to three
sets of ten on each side.

The bridge
Adopt the press-up position, resting on your elbows. Pull your stomach muscles in
tight towards your backbone, keeping your bottom down and your spine straight.
Hold this position for as long as you can, being careful not to arch your back. To
make it easier, drop to your knees. Keep looking down to the floor at all times.
Build up to thirty seconds and repeat three to five times.

Horizontal side support
Start by lying on your left side, resting on your left arm and with your legs extended
outwards and your right foot on top of the left. Slowly lift your pelvis off the floor
while supporting your weight on your left forearm and feet. Hold, keeping your
other arm by your side, for ten to fifteen seconds without letting your pelvis drop
down. Repeat five times on each side.

How did
it go?

Q   Are there any disciplines that focus on the waist?

A   *Pilates and yoga focus on the core muscles, i.e. the deep abdominal muscles that form your inner girdle. Belly dancing is all the rage these days. Have you ever seen an apple-shaped belly dancer? Or use a hoola hoop; post-natal women swear by them and it's far more challenging than it looks.*

Q   What can I do to fake a waist?

A   *Never wear baggy sack dresses or shifts. Instead, stick to dresses with waists and full skirts, and wrap-around tops that tie at the waist. And choose floaty fabrics, which can take inches off you. Deep V-necks, which draw the eye down and you 'in', are great. Thick belts, single-breasted jackets and wrap-around dresses will all nip your waist in and divide and separate. Also, boned corset tops (with optional whip) can look fantastic. Avoid double-breasted jackets or short bolero jackets that bulk you up.*

37

Skin from within

**With great nutrition and a little care, you can achieve
fabulous-looking skin in no time at all.**

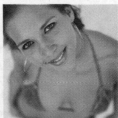

If you're anything like the rest of the population, how you look will be very important to you. We worry endlessly about the image we present to the world and a very important part of this is how our skin looks.

TUTTI FRUTTI

You probably don't need me to tell you that fruit and vegetables are the main ingredients to a healthy, youthful skin. The reason for this is that they contain lots of vitamins and minerals that perform an antioxidant function. Antioxidants mop up reactions caused by free radicals, which are unstable molecules created by such things as stress, pollution and certain foods. Free radicals sound like a new political party that we should all be voting for, but instead they're electrochemically unbalanced chemicals which ultimately can be the cause of degenerative diseases such as cancer and heart disease, not to mention premature ageing (which is where your skin comes in). The main antioxidant vitamins are vitamins A, C and E

Here's an idea for you...

Try to eat at least five portions of fruit and vegetables daily. And the more colours the better – try red peppers, yellow peppers, green peppers, red cabbage, sweet potatoes, etc. This way you can get enough antioxidants to help counter the effects of pollution. Be sure to buy organic though, as otherwise you could add to your toxic load!

together with the minerals selenium, manganese and zinc. Some B vitamins also have antioxidant properties together with some amino acids (building blocks for protein). Most of these important minerals can be found in a wholefood, fresh food diet.

Berries and fruits and vegetables with red, purple and blue colouring are particularly good because they're stuffed with antioxidants and contain a group of flavonoids called anthocyanidins, thought to be much more powerful than vitamin E. Antioxidants sometimes work together. For example, vitamins C and E work together – vitamin C allows vitamin E to be recycled in the body so that it can carry on working longer.

WATER YOUR FACE DAILY

Drinking pure, fresh water flushes toxins through your system and hydrates cells carrying essential nutrients to every part of your body. I probably didn't need to tell you that either. Aim to drink about 2 litres (3.5 pints) daily. Don't overdo it though or you could end up flushing minerals out of your system, especially if you're gulping rather than sipping.

FAT FACE!

The other essential ingredient to healthy skin is fat. Not any old fat, but essential fatty acids (EFAs). One group of EFAs is especially important: omega-3. EFAs work as a kind of waterproofer because they stop fluids escaping from your body's cells. In this way, your skin is kept plumped up and moisturised. Do an experiment – take a good quality fish oil supplement for three months (or flax seed if you're vegetarian) and note the quality of skin on the back of your hands. You'll notice that they're better moisturised!

You should also decrease the amount of saturated and processed fats in your diet, as these compete with the good fats and make their job more difficult. In general, the fresher the food and the more unprocessed it is, the wider the vitamin and mineral range and the more good it will do your skin!

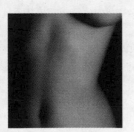 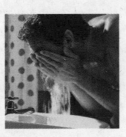

'All the beauty in the world, 'tis but skin deep.'
RALPH VENNING

Defining idea...

How did
it go?

Q **If fruit is so important for my skin, when can I fit in eating more fruit during the day?**

A *A great time to load up the fruit content is with your morning breakfast. I load up fruit on my morning oats – I tend to buy packs of blueberries, strawberries and raspberries. Make sure you wash soft fruit well as it's particularly bad for pesticide residues. You can buy frozen berries in most supermarkets and these are great for getting your flavonoids. You can, of course, snack on fruit at any time of the day – my favourite snack is an apple with a few nuts and seeds.*

Q **If I'm going to eat all these vegetables, I'm going to be doing a lot of chopping and preparing. Any tips to make this easier?**

A *I find that if I buy all my food supplies on Saturday and use Sunday for preparation, it's a lot easier for me to be ready for my week. Chop up all your main salad ingredients, such as red peppers, spring onion, grated carrot, salad leaves, and put them in ziplock bags, making sure that all the air is out (a little squeeze of lemon juice helps keep them fresh). Although not perfect from a purist's point of view because it's always best to chop vegetables as near to when you're going to eat them as possible, but in my view it's better to do something rather than nothing and this is a great way to cut down on preparation time.*

38

The beautiful and the bad

Seems as if only models and rock stars get good sex? Insecurity eats away at desire and anyone can have a hang-up.

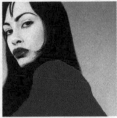

Don't let pictures of the beautiful and famous make you feel inadequate. Actually the top performers, models and stars probably feel more insecure than you do.

Beautiful women are held up as an ideal and yet top models, stars and performers suffer more than you think. They seem to have it all – looks, public adoration, money – but the cult of celebrity often makes people more insecure. Success is fleeting and many stars are anxious about losing their status or plagued with self-doubt and addictions. Jib Fowles did a study in *Starstruck: Celebrity Performers and the American Public* which showed that celebrities are four times more likely to kill themselves than the average person.

And it's not just the pressures of fame. Even the most beautiful women can have problems feeling confident. Halle Berry is a former Miss Teen All America, was the runner-up to Miss USA and has been voted onto *People* magazine's Most Beautiful People list nine times: oh, and she's also an Oscar winner. Despite all this, she

163

Here's an idea for you...

Get some glamorous photographs taken of you (if necessary by a professional) and keep a few of them, framed, in your bedroom. This is to remind you that you are sexy, and the better the photo the more confidence you'll feel. After all, glam shots in magazines are hardly simple snapshots!

recently announced that she is very insecure about both her physical appearance and her acting. On Femalefirst.com she said, about those who pay her compliments: 'If they really knew me, they'd realise I'm far from secure about my looks.' Knowing that such a successful, talented, good-looking woman is plagued by self-doubts should convince you that beauty is skin deep. There's no point in thinking that you would feel/be sexier if you looked differently; confidence comes from within.

Similarly, Madonna, who is perhaps the most media-savvy female performer ever, has admitted, 'I think my biggest flaw is my insecurity...I'm plagued with insecurities 24-7.' In *Madonna: An Intimate Biography*, J Randy Taraborrelli quotes dancer Sallim Gauwloos who appeared in the movie *In Bed with Madonna*: 'But she was very, very insecure, especially with other women. We would have parties, and there would never be beautiful women invited. Only guys. She would freak out if there was someone in the room more beautiful than her.' Clearly, public persona and how stars really feel are two different things. Lesson learnt – the grass is not greener on the other side.

One of the first supermodels of the late 70s, Gia Carangi, became a *Vogue* cover girl at eighteen and partied at New York's legendary Studio 54 with rock stars and royalty, but her spiralling

You know you want to, so be adventurous and turn to IDEA 33, *Let yourself go.*

Try another idea...

fame left her unable to live up to her public image. By twenty-six she became one of the first American women to die of AIDS: the biography of her life, *Thing of Beauty*, is not a pretty story.

Many regular women feel intimidated when they see airbrushed, perfect images of women in the media. A 2003 *Daily Mail* survey in the UK found only 3% of women were happy with their size; 25% of all women in the UK are on a diet at any one time, although around half of them are not even clinically overweight. In *The Body Project: An Intimate History of American Girls*, Joan Jacobs Brumberg says that girls' identities these days 'revolve around the body rather than the mind, heart, or soul'. We are just obsessed with how we look and having all this angst is a terrible burden on our sex lives.

In *Hot Monogamy* Dr Patricia Love uses research that shows women who have a negative body image are 'less interested in making love...more restricted in their range of sexual activities, and have more difficulty becoming aroused and reaching orgasm'. You have to feel sexy to have a better love life, rather than focusing on how you look. If you like, you can continue to feel down on yourself but it's better not to waste all that energy: concentrate instead on getting that orgasm high.

'A sex symbol becomes a thing. I hate being a thing.'
MARILYN MONROE

Defining idea...

How did it go?

Q   **There's always been a Lillie Langtry type. Why all this focus on pretty women in the media?**

A   *True, but today weight loss is a $50 billion per year industry in the US and the ideal of what we should look like is getting positively gaunt. As journalist Hazel Croft says: 'In the 1950s models weighed 8% less than the average woman. In the 1990s models weighed 23% less. That makes models thinner than some 95% of the population.' The difference between the ideal and the reality has never been further apart. Today there's so much more focus on how we look, people pierce their bodies, sculpt them with exercise and are increasingly turning to cosmetic surgery. But what do they actually achieve by doing all this?*

Q   **Even knowing the insecurities of people like Victoria Beckham doesn't stop me from feeling jealous. Am I alone?**

A   *No...there's a lot of it about. In a Nerve.com essay Lisa Gabriele is somewhat envious of Paris Hilton: 'She's so thin and pliable, she should register her body as a font.' If the overwhelming majority of us feel our bodies leave a lot to be desired, we're being our own worst enemies. Sex is one way we can learn to feel good about ourselves. Try simply spending time naked too; you need to get comfortable in your own skin.*

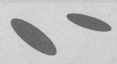

39

Back beauty

If you've never given your back a second thought, now's the time to make up for the neglect.

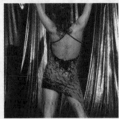

Do you only consider your back when summer arrives and it's suddenly on display or you're required to wear a strappy frock to a do? Suddenly you'll yearn for a flawless back and the firm, sinewy muscles of a ballet dancer.

If you're one of the 80% who suffer from back pain, you probably curse your back on a daily basis. We're told that 90% of back pain is postural, common culprits being carrying too much, slinging heavy handbags over our shoulders, slumping at work and spending hours in the car. Plus we have to lug our head around too, of course, which is no mean feat considering it weighs about 5–6 kg.

Try the following and give your back the attention it deserves:

Tense shoulders? Sore back? Try an aromatherapy bath. Add a few drops of Scotch pine, which is warming and good for sore muscles, or clary sage, which has anti-inflammatory properties.

TONE IT

Disciplines such as swimming (backstroke), Pilates and yoga are fantastic routes to a long, slender back and shoulders. Also, try the Alexander Technique, a postural alignment method of adding inches to your height.

Rowing is another excellent back firmer. Try this rowing-based exercise:

1. Hook a resistance band up to a heavy object such as a table leg; attach it three quarters of the way down the leg towards the floor.

2. Do a few stretches to warm up.

3. Stand with your feet hip-width apart, a few feet away from the table. Bend your knees into a half squat with your hips behind you and lean forwards, keeping your back straight and your head in line with your spine.

4. Take hold of the resistance band with both hands (palms facing). You should feel a stretch along the side of your body.

5. Keeping your back, legs and hips in the same position, exhale and bend your arms to pull the band towards your ribcage, making sure your elbows stay close to your body. Then, gently return to the starting position, making sure you maintain the tension in the band.

6. Repeat the move fifteen times, building up to two sets of repetitions.

7. Stretch afterwards. Standing a few feet away from a table or chair, bend your knees into a semi-squat and lean forwards, placing your hands, shoulder-width apart on the table or back of the chair. Step backwards and lean forwards so that your back and head are in line with your shoulders and arms. Hold for twenty seconds; make sure your knees are bent and your back isn't arched.

'Good shoulders and a long waist are the most necessary when it comes to wearing clothes.'
OLEG CASSINI

Defining idea...

FIRM UP THOSE SHOULDERS

Try this move, which targets your deltoids, the muscles that run from your collarbone at the front and each shoulder blade at the back, covering your shoulder and attaching at the back of your upper arms. All you need is a light chair that you can pick up without straining. Aim for a set of six repetitions, three times a week.

1. Stand with your feet hip-width apart and close to the chair. Viewed from the side, there should be a straight line from your ear to your shoulders, hips, knees and ankles.

2. Breathing in, bend your knees and push your hips out behind you as if you're about to sit down. Keeping your arms shoulder-width apart, gently take hold of the sides of the chair. Focus your attention on the chair.

169

3. As you breathe out, lift the chair to shoulder height, keeping your arms shoulder-width apart. Keep your shoulders down, your chin tucked in, your spine nice and long and your abs tight. Tuck your pelvis slightly under and hold this position for three to five seconds without holding your breath.

4. Gently lower the chair and return to the starting position.

CLEAR UP A SPOTTY BACK

Spots can ruin the effect of any strappy number. Keep the spotty area thoroughly clean, change your towels and bedlinen at least twice a week and cleanse your back at least once a day.

When you're cleansing your back, the key is to slough off the dead skin cells that cause blocked pores and spots. Apply a good-quality – ideally medicated – cleanser using your fingertips, then remove it with a muslin cloth. Try tea tree oil too; it has good antibacterial action, so either dab some on the spots themselves or add six to ten drops to a warm bath and lie back in the water for up to ten minutes. Don't use it with soap – which may interfere with its healing properties.

The back's a difficult area to reach yourself so you may want to invest in a salon treatment; the Guinot back cathiodermie treatment uses a combination of mild electrical current and Guinot gels and creams to revitalise the skin. Also, consider a visit to your doctor, as spots on your back may be the result of a hormonal imbalance.

Q I'm a bit ungainly. How can I stand more elegantly?

A Stand so that your weight is evenly balanced between both feet. Brace your abdominal muscles, pull in your stomach and keep your buttocks very gently squeezed. Keep your knees soft and lengthen your spine; imagine you've a piece of string running through it that's pulling you upwards. Keep your chin parallel to the floor and pull your shoulders back and downwards.

Q I often wake up with backache. Any tips?

A A bad bed and poor sleeping posture can pull your spine out of alignment. Choose a medium firm mattress and invest in a good bed. You'll only find out if it's supportive by road-testing it so lie down and slide your hand under the small of your back. If there's a large gap between the bed and your back the bed's too hard. If there's no gap or only a small one, the bed's too soft. Make sure your pillows are supportive and keep your head in line with the rest of your spine. Sleep with your head and neck – but not your shoulders – on the pillow. Don't use too many pillows or your head will be pushed up too high.

How did
it go?

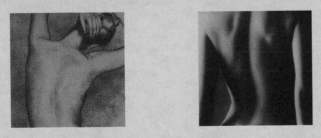

171

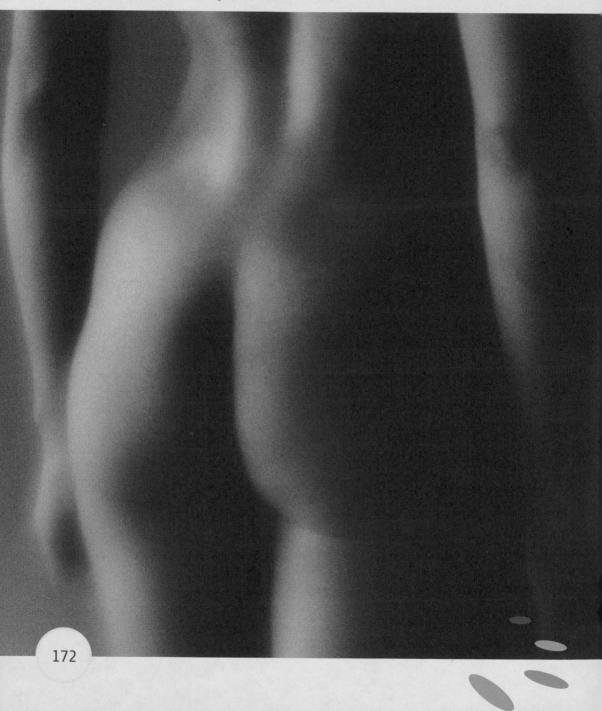

40

Bottom's Up

Celebrate your curves. Having cellulite – as nearly nine out of ten women do – doesn't mean you can't feel gorgeous. Try some bottom pampering today.

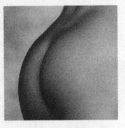

The word cellulite was first coined back in the 70s, but it's no modern affliction.

Just think of those Rubenesque lovelies, writhing about in the altogether. They'd never make the cover of today's *Vogue*, yet in their era they were considered the epitome of voluptuous sexiness.

Fashion has changed, and back in the days of yore, fatness (for that's essentially what cellulite is – body fat) would have been synonymous with wealth. Nowadays the smaller your thighs, the bigger your wallet. Women dread surplus pounds, aspiring instead to a neat peachy behind and racehorse legs. And cellulite, which becomes worse as you get older, is viewed as a sort of degenerative disease.

Face it. You know the horror you feel when you cross your legs and the orange peel bulges out. It's like viewing your first wrinkle or stretch mark. Somehow it's the beginning of the end.

The truth is cellulite is just part of being a woman – 85–95% of us fall prey to it, including the world's most glamorous models and actresses.

Here's an idea for you...

Toning up your behind doesn't have to be a full-time occupation. Try this tiny bum-firming move which you can do anywhere. Raise one foot off the floor and kick it back behind you in tiny pulse-moves. Aim for 15 repetitions two or three times a day.

There's nothing disease-like about it either: it's surplus fat held together by skin cells that have lost their elasticity. And it lurks about the areas of a woman's body that are designed to lay down fat – backs of thighs, bottoms, tummies, even your upper arms. The result? Fat cells squishing upwards against your skin and causing a cottage cheese effect – like stuffing bursting out of an old cushion.

That's not to say you have to embrace cellulite as part of your femaleness (that's why we've written this book, after all). But before you get stressed, depressed and obsessed about the cellulitey bits, take a moment here to get a perspective, and to celebrate your curves.

A friend's husband once took a mould of her behind, which was, refreshingly, generously proportioned. He gave it to her as an anniversary present – a wonderful pumpkin of a bottom cast in bronze.

So the first lesson is 'remember, men love curves'. In fact men particularly love fleshy bottoms when they're paired with a small waist; studies show a waist/hip ratio of 0.7 is the magic formula most likely to get a man's pulse racing.

Don't forget too that your curves are there for a reason: making babies, having babies, feeding babies, filling out bikinis/ridiculously expensive undies, that sort of thing.

Your curves also give *you* pleasure. Legs, bottoms, thighs, tummies – they're all part of your healthy, functioning, living, breathing body. So think of a slightly dimply bottom as a sign of a rich, happy and fulfilling life.

Oh, and a spongy bottom is also handy at weddings and on bikes; pews and saddles can be so uncomfortable.

'*Everything has its beauty, but not everyone sees it.*'
CONFUCIUS

Defining
idea...

So let's start by nipping that self-criticism in the bud. Time, instead, to celebrate that ass. Try some of these today:

■ Savour the good things about your bum and thighs – the excitement of slipping into new silky pants, that satisfying pain/exhilaration when you cycle up a hill, the sensation of rubbing lovely cream into your legs, someone else fondling your behind...

■ Every day, promise yourself you'll do something that makes you feel good about your body – have something really delicious to eat, treat yourself to a day at a spa, go for a swim, book a fantastic holiday. Doing something pleasurable can make you feel happy.

■ Stop buying clothes that don't fit but which you're aiming to 'diet into'. They make you feel worse about your body. Instead, buy yourself something big but gorgeous that you can wear now.

■ Make a mental list of your best bits – glossy hair, pretty feet, long, beautifully shaped fingernails, trim calves, firm boobs. Stop focusing on your shortcomings and acknowledge your glories.

■ Splash out on body treats: indulging really does boost your self-confidence – book a facial/manicure, buy new perfume, wallow in a luxurious, gorgeous smelling bath. Take pleasure in looking your best.

■ Start taking some exercise. It can boost your mood, improve your complexion, help you focus and give you confidence in your body.

How did it go?

Q   I'm bombarded with billboards featuring images of teenage girls with super-smooth bottoms. How can I possibly feel good about my own bum?

A   Invest in a beautiful coffee-table art book and peruse the images of real women that artists over the centuries have deemed beautiful – you'll find curves aplenty there. Visit galleries, muse over a Rodin sculpture. And think about your most attractive friends and colleagues. Do they have buttocks you could crack nuts with? Probably not. More likely they're confident, and exude joie de vivre. Remember there's more to beauty than the size and texture of your ass.

Q   That's all very well, but what about all those holiday snaps of me looking round and dimply? Not very good for my body image.

A   OK, so have a clearout. It's good therapy to get rid of old 'fat' photographs of you, which make you miserable. Instead collect pictures of yourself looking your best/slimmest/prettiest/happiest. It helps you realise you're a lot tastier than you give yourself credit for.

41

Points on posture

How you hold yourself can make you look and feel longer, leaner and more confident. Shoulders back now, ladies.

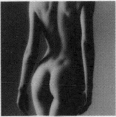

To improve your posture in days gone by you simply balanced a few books on your head and walked elegantly around a room. These days improving posture is an altogether more athletic pursuit.

The key to great posture is to stabilise your core, i.e. the muscles that run around your body – your natural corset if you like. Pilates is the ultimate tummy-flattening, posture-boosting discipline as it's based on firming precisely these muscles. Pilates can also be a great libido booster as strengthening your abs, back and pelvic floor can enhance sexual function and response.

Try the Pilates 'zip and hollow' method, an easy but effective posture booster. Whenever you zip or button up your trousers, pull in your pelvic floor muscles while you hollow your lower abdominals back towards your spine. That way you're working the deepest layer of abdominal muscles. You can do this exercise anywhere, in fact, and it's even more effective than sit-ups in terms of firming your tummy.

Been sitting down for too long? Counter bad posture with this exercise. Begin on all fours with your weight evenly distributed and your hands and knees shoulder-width apart. Pull your left knee towards your chest with your right hand, simultaneously curling your head towards your chest. Uncurl slowly, extending your left leg and right hand until they're horizontal to the floor; your back should be in a straight line. Repeat on the opposite side after placing your left knee and hand slightly forward of the starting position. Do five sequences; you should find you're moving across the floor.

STAND TALL

■ Imagine there's a string pulling you up from the centre of your head. Whether you're walking, sitting or standing, think tall and 'feel' that string gently pulling you up. Your stomach should be pressed flat.

■ Relax your shoulders down into your back. When they feel tight, raise them up to your ears, squeezing them up and together as hard as you can, as if you're doing an exaggerated shrug, then just drop them and feel the tension ease. Try squeezing your shoulder blades together behind you; it's a great way to keep your shoulders back.

■ Position your pelvis as neutral as possible and keep your waist long. Don't let your ribcage 'fall' into your hips.

■ When you stand, make sure you soften your knees. If you lock your legs, you'll end up arching your back and throwing the rest of your body out of line. Also, make sure you put equal weight on each foot. If you're standing with more weight on one foot or with one foot turned out you'll look crooked.

■ Keep your chin parallel to the floor.

SIT UP STRAIGHT

- Sit at the end of your chair and slouch
  completely. Draw yourself up and
  accentuate the curve of your back as far as
  possible. Hold for a few seconds and then release the position slightly (about ten
  degrees). This is a good sitting posture.
- Make sure your back is straight and your shoulders back. Your buttocks should
  touch the back of your chair. A small, rolled-up towel or a lumbar roll can be
  used to help you maintain the normal curves in your back.
- Distribute your body weight evenly on both hips.
- Bend your knees at a right angle, keeping them slightly higher than your hips.
  Keep your feet flat on the floor. If necessary, use a footrest or stool.
- Never cross your legs.
- Try to avoid sitting in the same position for more than thirty minutes.
- At work, adjust your chair height and workstation so you can sit up close to your
  computer screen and tilt it up at you. Rest your elbows and arms on your chair
  or desk, making sure you keep your shoulders relaxed.

'Taking joy in life is a woman's best cosmetic.'
ROSALIND RUSSELL, actress

Defining idea...

STRENGTHEN THOSE ABS

Start on your hands and knees. While exhaling raise your right arm and left leg until
they're level with your torso. Keep your hips even and look down so that your neck
is aligned. Contract your abs, but don't tuck your pelvis under or arch your back.
Pull in your pelvic floor muscles and pull your tummy button in towards your
backbone. Slowly return to the start and then repeat on the other side. Do two sets
of eight repetitions on each side.

How did it go?

Q   I sit at a desk all day and I know my posture suffers. How can I improve my working posture?

A   *Most of us go for hours at a time without moving, which puts a strain on our spines and causes us to slump. Even jobs that involve standing can ruin our posture. Make sure your ergonomics are correct at work. Get up every twenty minutes to stretch and change position. Stretch out your arms as if you were yawning and lean right back. Move your hands as far away as possible and hold the stretch for as long as you can. Repeat every twenty minutes or so.*

Q   What's the best posture to adopt when driving? I spend hours in the car each day.

A   *Make sure your lower back is supported and always push your buttocks right into the back of the seat. Move the seat close to the steering wheel to support the curve of your back. If necessary, use a back support such as a rolled-up towel. The seat should be close enough to allow your knees to bend while reaching the pedals. When resting, your knees should be at the same level or higher than your hips.*

42

Easy ways to lose a pound a week without trying too hard

Simple food swaps, cutting back on high-calorie treats and pushing yourself to be a little more active can help you achieve realistic, long-term weight loss. Mix and match these tips and you will look and feel slimmer with minimum effort.

There is always a less fattening choice of snack to be made, or a calorie-minimising way to cook. Take one of my favourite meals, the Caesar salad. It's a salad, so it must be good for you, right? Wrong!

Unfortunately, the Caesar salad has one of the most fattening dressings known to the hips, plus enough cheese and croutons to demand its own place setting at dinner. What can you do, apart from gaze at it longingly from across a crowded room? You can make a lighter version, that's what. Just replace the fried croutons

Here's an idea for you...

Chew sugar-free gum or clean your teeth after a meal or a snack. As well as cleaning your teeth and giving you sweet breath, it sends you a psychological message that you have finished eating and that it is time to do something else. Make a clean break when your meal ends so that you really know that it is over.

with baked ones, reduce the cheese drastically and go very light on the oil. There's always a solution, you see.

One of the best solutions to losing a little bit of weight every week is to make changes that are so simple, you'll barely notice them. It's safe and possible to lose half a kilo (a pound) a week if you shave 500 calories per day from your food intake (or expend it through activity). The maths behind this is that 3,500 calories equals half a kilo (a pound) of fat. So, divide 7 days into 3,500 and you get that magic 500 number. Do some more maths and you'll see that 500 g a week is 2 kg a month and 12 kg in six months. Get started with the following clever little ideas:

Say no to crisps

This is one of the most popular snacks, but a regular 40 g bag has around 200 calories and 10 g of fat. Even lighter versions come in at slightly over half that amount. So if you stopped having a bag each day at work, you'd save at least 500 calories a week.

Avoid large portions

A large burger, fries and fizzy drink will easily stack up to 1000 calories, if not slightly more. If you can't cut them out, at least opt for the regular or small sizes which will cut the calories in half.

Watch what you drink

On a night out, three 175 ml glasses of white wine will cost you nearly 400 calories. Three spritzers will be half that. A half pint of strong lager clocks up around 160 calories, while a half of ordinary strength is about 80 calories. Steer clear of cocktails too – a pina colada is easily 225 calories, while a vodka and slimline tonic is just 60.

On your bike

Eco-friendly, fun and jolly good exercise, an hour's cycling should take care of nearly 500 calories.

Sandwich swap

If you have a little low fat salad cream in your lunchtime sandwich instead of lashings of butter, you could save up to 500 calories during your working week.

Rethink your Saturday night take-away

Choose chicken chow mein and boiled rice over sweet and sour chicken and fried rice, you'll save around 500 calories.

Walk more

If you walk to work, the shops or just for fun (but at a reasonably brisk pace) you'll burn up around 250 calories an hour.

'Another good reducing exercise consists of placing both hands against the table edge and pushing back.'
ROBERT QUILLEN

Defining idea...

183

Wash the car

Save money and burn energy by valeting your car. Wash it, polish it and vacuum it inside and you'll use up a few hundred calories,

Have a skinnier coffee

You could save yourself 170 calories if you opted for a regular white coffee, made with skimmed milk, rather than a cappuccino made with full fat milk.

Party snacks

Think such small little nibbles don't count? If you had two tablespoons of tzatziki dip that would add up to around 40 calories. Two tablespoons of taramasalata, however, is 130 calories. Thick meat pate on French bread can cost you about 250 calories, whereas a small helping of smoked salmon on rye bread is a mere 130 calories. A cocktail sausage is around 70 calories. Wrap it in pastry and serve it as a sausage roll and you're looking at 200 calories.

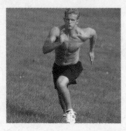
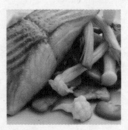
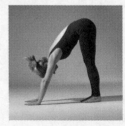

Q   **My weakness is cheese. How can I lose weight and still indulge?**

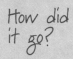

How did it go?

A   *Keep your portion sizes matchbox small and enjoy a delicious ripe piece of fruit with it. Some cheeses are also more heavyweight than others. Cheddar, for example, is around 124 calories per 30 g with around 10 g of fat. The same weight of camembert is about 90 calories with 7 g of fat, while feta is 75 calories and 6 g of fat. Check labels to make comparisons and the best choices. You could also try grating cheese to have on toast or a cracker rather than slicing it, so you still get the taste, only fewer calories.*

Q   **I'm too busy to walk or cycle, so I can't really burn up extra energy that way, can I?**

A   *Ultimately you're going to have to find a way to schedule some exercise into your life. You could start by breaking it down into smaller chunks. For example, if you took half an hour's walking a day as your target, you could break it down into three ten minute sessions, say a walk before breakfast, one at lunchtime and one in the evening. I don't think that's impossible for anyone.*

Q   **Does it help you lose weight if you don't eat after 6 p.m.?**

A   *There isn't a proven link between eating in the evening and gaining weight. You might eat more over dinner, especially if you eat out, but your metabolism isn't slowing down as dusk falls. It does when you're asleep though!*

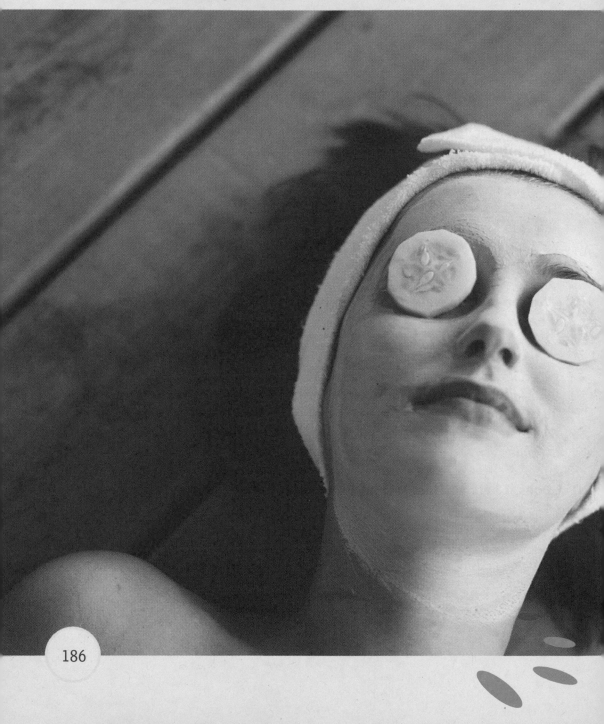

43

Clean, green beauty queen

**Cosmetics and toiletries are jaw-droppingly expensive –
for men and for women. So, take the downshifted option –
make your own!**

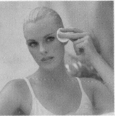

When you buy that expensive but oh-so-
pretty pot of cream, with all its beguiling
promises, you are paying for a dream wrapped up
in expensive advertising.

My mother always told me never to put anything on my skin that I wouldn't gladly put in my mouth. It's good advice, and makes you smell quite deliciously edible. The products we buy are cocktails of chemicals – even most of the products that trumpet how 'natural' they are in their advertising. Parabens and phthalates, which are potentially carcinogenic, are found in all manner of toiletries and cosmetics. Phthalates are often found in hairspray, perfume, and facial moisturisers, and parabens are present in many deodorants and toothpastes.

We absorb substances through our skin, so it makes sense to make those substances as natural as possible.

Here's an idea for you...

Who needs expensive bath products? You can make your own bath bombs with materials bought cheaply from the chemists. Mix together: 1/4 cup of baking soda, 1 tablespoon of ascorbic acid, 1 tablespoon of borax powder and 2 tablespoons of icing sugar. Add 2 tablespoons of sweet almond oil, together with fragranced oil. You can also add herbs from your garden. Press the mixture firmly into moulds – cheap flexible rubber ice cube moulds are ideal. After a couple of hours these can be turned out onto waxed paper to dry for a few days. Store the 'bombs' in a closed container. To use them, drop them into your bath water and watch them fizz!

FACE

Honey, raw egg and oatmeal mixed together makes a lovely face mask (or a manly facial scrub). If you are having trouble with spots and blemishes, add a drop of tea tree oil for its antiseptic properties – but be cautious when using oils because they are very strong and can cause irritation if you use too much.

Kaolin powder or fuller's earth (types of clay) can be mixed with strong herb 'tea' or a couple of drops of soothing oil, such as chamomile, to make a pore-tightening face mask. Leave it on until it dries, then have fun scaring the cat and generally 'cracking your face' before you rinse it off with water.

Yoghurt – natural, not fruity and bitty – makes a good cleanser for all skin types, and jojoba oil (a type of liquid wax) makes a great moisturiser.

Make a gentle facial scrub by mixing ground almonds with rose water. You can make your own rose water by steeping rose petals in water in a jar on a sunny windowsill for a day or so (no longer or it will grow interesting fur; not something you would want to spread on your face!), and then adding a couple of drops of rose oil and a few fresh finely chopped petals.

HAIR

Chamomile is well known as a rinse for bringing out highlights in blonde hair. Just make a strong 'tea' and use it as a last rinse after washing your hair. Rhubarb stems can be boiled and the liquor used to lighten hair. Wash your hair and comb through the liquid (made by boiling two sticks of chopped rhubarb in a pan of water until it turns to mush, then straining it). Leave it in for half an hour and then rinse.

Sage 'tea' can be used as a final rinse for dark hair, and 1 teaspoon of cider vinegar added to final rinsing water is good for making any shade of hair silky. Raw eggs, whisked in a jug, make a strange but effective conditioner for supple, shiny hair – just don't rinse with hot water or you'll end up covered in scrambled egg.

I'm tired of all this nonsense about beauty being only skin-deep. That's deep enough. What do you want, an adorable pancreas?
JEAN KERR, author and playwright

Defining idea...

BODIES

Ground rock salt or sugar makes a wonderful and invigorating body and foot scrub. Add olive oil and a few drops of essential oil according to your mood, and even a few fresh chopped herb leaves such as mint or lemon verbena. Just scrub and rinse for baby soft skin!

BATHS

Make a fragrant bath without getting bits stuck all over your body by simmering a handful of herbs or flowers in water for about 15 minutes. Leave the liquid to cool and sieve it before adding it to your bath. Alternatively, make mixtures of dried or fresh herbs and put them in small home-made drawstring muslin bags (Cut a circle of muslin and stitch round the edge – put the herbs in and pull the thread tight.) Hang them under the running bath water.

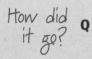

Q   I'd like to make my own cosmetics because I'm against animal testing, but how can I be sure that the products I make are safe?

A   Firstly, use the 'can I eat it?' test – that is, make toiletries from food substances. You can also do a patch test on your own skin. Rub a small amount of the cosmetic preparation you have made onto a small patch of your own skin and leave it overnight. The inner elbow is a good place because the skin is quite sensitive and it can be hidden if it goes blotchy! If all goes well and you do not have a reaction, go ahead and use your 'product'.

Q   There are loads of ideas I'd like to try, but what can I store the goodies I make in?

A   Well, you can reduce the amount of rubbish sent to the landfill site by reusing tubs and bottles you have bought, and friends save for you. I also buy pretty glass bottles and jars from junk shops. Make small quantities, and store your products in the fridge if possible, as they will last longer. Remember, cosmetic firms put preservatives into their products to make them last and you do not.

44

Hands-on treatments

Your hands speak volumes about your toilette. If you can't stretch to salon manicures, there are easy ways to titivate your nails on the cheap.

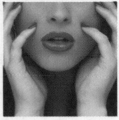

Think of your nails as the icing on a cake — the finishing touch to your outfit, shoes, hair and make-up. A neatly manicured set says you're well groomed and glamorous.

The first steps to gorgeous hands are to wash and dry them regularly and to always use hand cream. Keep a jar by every sink in your house plus one in your handbag. Okay, most women are meticulous about hygiene and we don't need reminding to wash our hands after using the loo. However, the more you do it the better. Interestingly, one US study found that if you wash your hands five times a day you could dramatically slash your risk of catching germs and getting ill. It was based on a two-and-a-half year hand-washing programme conducted by the navy. Another reason why everyone loves a sailor!

Here's an idea for you...

To calm yourself in moments of stress and to relieve headaches and any tension in your neck and shoulders, apply pressure to the acupoint between your thumb and first finger (to find it, feel for the muscle that you feel when you press your thumb and index finger together). Press for one second, then 'pump' for a minute.

Don't underestimate the protective powers of a pair of Marigolds. Always use rubber gloves when washing up. Also, use them when cleaning as household-cleaning products can make your skin dry and your nails dry and brittle.

A nightly trick to soften hands is to smother Vaseline, or petroleum jelly, into your nails, which will have a dramatic effect on taming your cuticles. For best results wear cotton gloves to bed afterwards and you'll wake with beautifully soft hands.

You can eat your way to better nails, too, say the experts. The best foods for nails include plenty of protein (fish, meat, soya, tofu, eggs) to help them grow and prevent those white lines from appearing across them. And B vitamins, found in eggs, seafood and root vegetables, are a good way to keep nasty ridges at bay. Eat plenty of fish, fish oils and seeds, which are all rich in essential fatty acids that help nourish nails. Foods rich in zinc, such as seafood, lean meat and wholegrains, help prevent white spots. Brittle nails? You'll need to eat lots of calcium and vitamin-A foods such as carrots, peaches, leafy vegetables and tinned fish, which are great for strengthening dry nails.

Treat yourself to a home manicure every week or two and save the real thing for special occasions. Remove old polish and then shape each nail with an emery board (nail files are too severe). Don't saw away at your nails or you'll break them. Instead, use light strokes from the edges towards the centre. Massage your cuticles with cuticle cream or add a few drops of cuticle massage oil to a bowl of warm water. Soak your cuticles for five minutes, then push them back using a cuticle stick. Wash your hands, then apply a protective base coat of clear varnish to your nails, followed by a coat or two of colour. Leave your hands for twenty minutes or so to avoid smudging them, then add a sealing topcoat.

Don't forget to apply sunscreen on your hands. We rarely think about protecting our hands from the sun because we don't often burn there, but hands will give away your age better than any other part of your body and can even add a few cruel years too, so look after them. I once worked with a PR for a beauty company. She was based in LA and wore taupe leather gloves everywhere she went to protect her skin. She may have had a touch of the Howard Hughes about her, but it worked and she had the hands of a twelve year old.

'Without grace, beauty is an unbaited hook.'
FRENCH PROVERB

Defining idea...

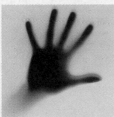

How did it go?

Q **What can I do to minimise my huge hands?**

A *Try wearing billowy sleeves, which make arms and hands look daintier. Huge jewellery, such as chunky gold or silver bangles and elaborate rings, can make hands and fingers look smaller. Keeping hands exfoliated and moisturised can make them seem more feminine.*

Q **I have yellowing nails. What can I do to whiten them?**

A *Wearing nail varnish regularly can cause yellowing nails, so go au naturel at least one or two days each week, which will bring the natural pink colour back in no time. Also, scrub your nails regularly to clean them and try soaking them in lemon juice for a few minutes, which can remove stains without drying your skin.*

Q **What's a cheap way to pamper my hands without getting a manicure?**

A *Once a week apply a moisturising face pack to your hands and leave for ten or fifteen minutes. Then rinse it off and give your hands a massage with some lovely rich gooey handcream or a natural oil such as almond or grapeseed.*

45

Up in arms

The rebellion against crinkly upper arms starts here. Yes, you *can* wear sleeveless dresses again.

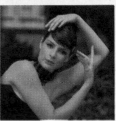

As if cellulite on the nether regions wasn't enough, some of us have got it on the backs of our arms too. But it doesn't have to stay there, there's a lot you can do to shift it — without even leaving your sofa.

A much smaller percentage of women have cellulite on their upper arms compared to those who get it on their thighs and bottoms, but for those who do it's just as annoying and confidence-denting as getting it anywhere else – if not more so. Your arms are so much more visible, and most people cursed with crepey skin here would give their right arm (well that's one way of getting shot of it) to be cellulite-free. Who wants to wear long sleeves all summer and never get to slink around in a strappy evening dress?

Just like the hips and bottom, women are genetically predisposed to store fat on their upper arms. Fat accumulation here also tends to get worse the older we get. You've heard the one about women over forty being advised not to wave anyone goodbye while wearing a sleeveless dress? Batwings, bingo wings or whatever other unflattering name you want to give them, it's this wobbly excess flesh that attracts cellulite like wasps to a jar of jam.

Here's an idea for you... **Look for dresses with wispy chiffon sleeves – the sheer fabric will give your arms just enough camouflage but will still look glamorous and sexy.**

It's possible to be quite slim and still have wobbly upper arms, so it's not only those who are carrying excess weight that are vulnerable – but the first thing to do to get rid of cellulite here is to shed the pounds if you're over your ideal weight. If you're prone to cellulite in this area you can't afford to carry excess baggage.

Not waving but toning

The next thing to do is to really tone up your upper arms – it can take years off your overall appearance. Madonna and Jerry Hall have reached the flabby arm age but you don't see them waving batwings at their fans. If they can do it, so can you. You don't need a personal trainer or any expensive equipment either.

Think about the general exercise you're doing at the moment – how much of it involves your upper arms? Maybe you're running and cycling, but you're not doing much for your upper body. Try swimming – both front crawl and breaststroke will help you trim down and sculpt upper arms. Both use powerful tricep movements, and pushing against the water adds resistance.

If you're a walker, don't just shove your hands in your pockets, buy a couple of Nordic walking poles (available from sports shops) and give your arms a workout as well as your legs. Nordic walking, during which you swing your poles rhythmically to help you along, really uses the muscles on the backs of the arms *and* burns extra calories.

Best home exercise: tricep dips

The tricep dip is a simple exercise to tone up flabby skin on the underside of the arms and help diminish cellulite.

- Sit on a dining chair, bench or even the side of bath, gripping the edge of the seat/bath or placing your palms flat down on the surface, close to your body.

'Time may be a great healer, but it's a lousy beautician.'
ANON

Defining idea...

- Put your legs out in front with your feet flat on the floor – the further away your feet are the more you will work your triceps.

- Using your arms to support yourself, ease your body forwards and drop your bottom almost to the floor, then return to your starting position.

- Repeat 10–20 times, rest and then do another set. Do as many sets as you can – at least three or four – and nearly every day of the week if possible. It only takes a matter of minutes and the more you do the quicker the results.

Roll your sleeves up

You may be able to improve the look of the back of cellulitey arms by self-massage. As it's a small area it doesn't take long and you don't have to take your clothes off, so you could do it any time you've got a spare few minutes. Buy some massage oil or rich body lotion and use firm, circular movements and some gentle kneading.

Is cosmetic surgery an option?

Yes, but it's a drastic measure and will leave scars on the underside of your upper arms, sometimes reaching as far down as the elbow. It's sometimes considered for those who have lost a lot of weight quickly and are left with loose skin that no amount of arm exercises seems to shift completely.

How did it go?

Q **Does dry skin brushing help cellulite on the arms like it does on the thighs?**

A *Yes, and, as you would on your lower body, you should brush in the direction of the heart to stimulate lymphatic drainage – so brush from the elbow to the armpit.*

Q **I don't have cellulite on the back of my arms but I've got lots of tiny bumps like minute pimples – they make my arms feel really rough. Are they the beginnings of cellulite? And how can I get rid of them?**

A *This is not the beginnings of cellulite, it's a common complaint and is likely to be caused by the skin becoming slightly dry, particularly in winter when we spend most of our time in centrally heated environments. Give the area a good exfoliation with a body scrub every time you're in the bath or shower to encourage cell turnover, then afterwards massage with a heavy moisturiser, such as those formulated for dry skin.*

Q **I hardly have time for exercise. Have you got any tips how I can fit this in to my busy day?**

A *Who cleans your windows? Think twice before you pay a window cleaner. It's great exercise for the upper arms, so get the Windolene out and save yourself some money. If you do it once a week you'll get a good workout and have the cleanest windows in the street. Or keep a set of hand weights next to the sofa. Every time you sit down to watch the news or your favourite soap, use them to trim your triceps.*

198

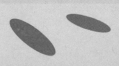

46

Spa therapy

The first time I went to a spa, I was a bit overwhelmed. I walked in and came across two naked women frolicking on a swing, legs akimbo. I prayed I wasn't expected to join in.

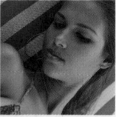

Now I've realised this experience was the exception rather than the rule. The earliest spas may have been peopled by naked nymphs fondling conches, but not any more.

These days, the best spas are stress-free havens that smell divine, with softly spoken therapists, subdued lighting and warbly music. The meals are generous, wine isn't a dirty word, and far from licensing nudity, everything is done to protect your modesty.

Spas are wonderful places – little fantasy worlds of sheer indulgence, totally devoted to serenity, peace and quiet. For that reason, don't bring your mobile phone or talk loudly. They can be a little reminiscent of that 60s show *The Prisoner* – lots of people walking about looking dazed (stunned into silence by the blissful massages). Plus the white fluffy robes can make you feel a number, not a name – almost like you're in a hospital ward. Still, for a girly treat, hen do or solo sojourn there's nothing like an afternoon in a spa for brushing away those cobwebs and making you feel all woman again.

Here's an idea for you...

Plan your own pamper party. Get the girls over, get into your dressing gowns, and experiment with make-up, nail colours, hair dos. Swap any unopened bottles of perfume or lipsticks that just aren't 'you'. You may find a few bargains. Add a few bottles of bubbly and some posh chocs and you'll be in heaven.

Personally I prefer hotels with fantastic spas – somewhere you can slip from your treatment room to the bar, and have an excuse to get out of the bathrobe and into heels come dusk. Preferably with acres of grounds, fitness classes and a mouth-watering menu. And with the odd finishing touch – such as playrooms/ nannies/crèches, grape peelers, that sort of thing.

If you're new to spas, here are a few treatments/disciplines you may want to try – and what they can do for you:

ACUPUNCTURE

An ancient Chinese therapy which involves placing tiny needles in certain points in the body – its channels of energy – to boost the flow of that energy (known as chi), in order to restore the body's balance and encourage the body to heal itself. Used to beat back and joint pain, digestive problems, skin disorders, anxiety and insomnia, depression, menstrual problems.

REFLEXOLOGY

Diagnostic massage of the feet which uses acupoints to re-energise the body and encourage healing. The therapist gently manipulates points in your feet to treat areas of weakness. Wonderfully relaxing. Used to beat stress, anxiety, sleep disorders, back and neck pain, hormonal imbalances, digestive disorders, migraine.

AYURVEDA

A 5,000-year-old Indian healing system which involves analysis of your lifestyle and body type – after which you're classified into either vata, pitta and kapha metabolic type. Treatment depends on your individual type, and usually includes various methods such as herbs, oils, dietary advice, yoga, massage, meditation. Often used for allergies, skin problems, digestive disorders, gynaecological complaints.

LA STONE THERAPY

An ancient healing treatment, which involves heated and cool stones being placed along the spine, then gently massaged over the body to relax the tissues. The stones are said to warm the muscles of your back, and soothe stresses and strains. Good for sore muscles, anxiety, neck and back pain.

CACI

Dubbed the 'non-surgical face lift', this is said to firm the skin using the transmission of tiny electrical impulses and signals to stimulate muscle tone and enhance skin tissue. A course of ten sessions is usually recommended, but after just one session you really can look brighter, fresher, less droopy!

OXYGEN FACIAL

This involves the usual cleansing, firming and moisturising you get during a facial, and the smothering of lovely unguents. But the unique selling point is the application of rejuvenating oxygen deep into the skin using a no-needle injection –

or pressurised jet. Recommended to help boost elasticity, help reduce fine lines, it's good for smokers' skin and acne, and results can be dramatic.

FOUR HANDS MASSAGE

A sublime and very, er, thorough massage, administered by not one but two therapists using a combination of short, deep and long sweeping strokes to iron out those knots. Slightly unorthodox as it may initially seem, it's wonderfully synchronised, intense and pleasurable, and deeply relaxing. Great for sleep problems, sore muscles, anxiety, stress.

'It is impossible to overdo luxury.'
FRENCH PROVERB

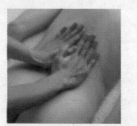 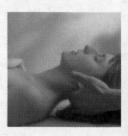

Q **I like the thought of a spa, but I'm not sure about baring my all. Do many treatments require nudity?**

How did it go?

A *Not all. Therapies such as shiatsu, Indian head massage and reflexology are performed fully clothed. But if you are required to disrobe, there are usually pairs of fetching paper pants you can pop on for modesty's sake. Besides, the therapist should leave the room while you undress, the lights should be dimmed and you should be able to cover yourself with towels. There shouldn't be a video recorder filming, an audience, that sort of thing.*

Q **What should I do about tipping?**

A *The usual tip is about 10–15% of the bill, the same as for hairdressers. You can either hand it to your therapist after your treatment, or add it to the final bill – it's up to you. Don't feel you have too; if it wasn't that great, don't bother.*

Q **I really prefer to lie down and close my eyes during a treatment rather than chat to the therapist. How can I drop a subtle hint?**

A *Your therapist will be used to people dropping off, so won't be offended. Start the treatment by telling her (or him) about any niggles, concerns, whether you'd like firmer pressure on your back and shoulder, that sort of thing. Then when she gets to work, close your eyes say something like, 'do excuse me if I drift off. I usually do during massages'. She'll get the picture. (Incidentally, if you'd prefer a same-sex therapist, request one when booking your treatment.)*

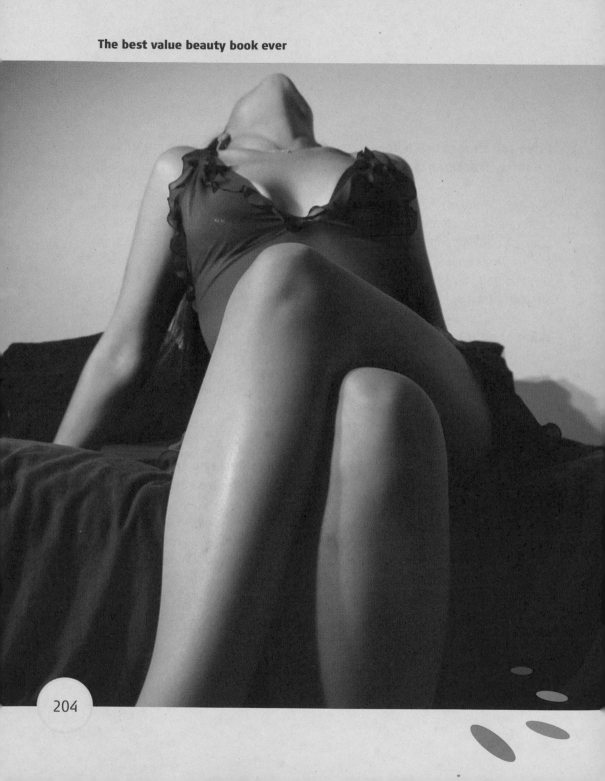

47

Sexual confidence

What is sexual confidence? And how do you get your hands on some?

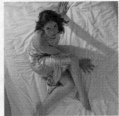

If you're uptight about sex, insecure about your body or just plain worried that you're not very good at it, then building sexual confidence is a prerequisite to enjoying yourself.

What factor most affects your ability to have a brilliant sex life? A great body? A fabulous lover? A bendy body? If you've got all these – bully for you. Even so, without one all-important element, your sex life is still likely to be ho-hum rather than bloody fantastic. You must have sexual confidence.

WHAT MIGHT WORK

This is where my feminist principles go out of the window. Truth is, if you're feeling lacklustre about your appearance – male or female – it's very unlikely you're having a great sex life. Forget *cherchez la femme*, or *cherchez l'homme* for that matter. I say, *cherchez le diet*. A dramatic weight loss in a long-term partner should always be viewed with terrific suspicion. If your lover loses stones and your love life is less than sparkling, you'd better start improving your bedroom skills because their sexual confidence is going to go sky high and when that happens, thrilling sex is never far away. With or without you.

Here's an idea for you...

Work on feeling more sexual every day. Think of yourself as a powerfully sexual person. Look for opportunities to make life more sensual. Flirt.

On the other hand, if you've been feeling less like sex, ask yourself whether being 5 kg lighter would make a difference to your libido. If it would, then diet. The most successful diet I've come across in recent years is the South Beach Diet by Dr Arthur Agatston. It's healthy and it works.

And this is where I go the whole nine yards and tear up my ticket as a card-carrying feminist. I would love to write with bravado that if you think having bigger/firmer/smaller boobs would improve your sex life you're frankly bonkers. But I'm not sure. As a child, I smashed my teeth falling off a bike. I had bad veneers fitted to replace them. As I proceeded through my twenties, I became self-conscious about smiling and eventually even about talking, so I had new, more expensive dental work and felt more confident. Have I the right to sneer at those who think fiddling with their body parts will make a difference to their sexual confidence? No. But beware. Your goal is sexual confidence. If it's your partner who wants you to have surgery, you won't gain sexual confidence. And if you've had a boob job already, I very much doubt that having smoother thighs will make the difference. These are distractions, and your relationship with either your partner or yourself is at fault. Spend your money on therapy or a self-esteem course instead.

Finally, if you're a bloke, please don't waste your money on penis-enhancing aids that you see in magazines. I'd like to say to you that women don't worry about size, but I can't as they do. But it would be an unusual woman who chucked a bloke because his penis didn't live up to her previous lover's penis. If your penis is smaller than average – anything less than five inches erect – you'll have to be kinder, smarter, funnier and better in bed than other men. Unfair I know, but life isn't fair.

Some penis pumps will work temporarily. There are apparently two operations that can increase either the girth or the length of the penis that actually work. They also can cause problems, and if the penis-lengthening operation goes wrong, you actually end up with a shorter penis. I jest not.

SO WHAT DOES WORK?

- **Change your perception.** Do what it takes to feel as attractive as you can. Then start talking yourself up: 'I'm happy', 'I look great', 'I'm gorgeous.' Repeat your affirmations twenty times daily.

- **Look in a mirror.** As we get older or busier, we spend less time looking in the mirror and try to pretend our body just isn't there. A mistake. Buy a full-length mirror. Look at yourself naked. Look at yourself dressed. Spend time preening. Throw out everything that doesn't make you feel great and look brilliant. If that leaves you with three items of clothing, so be it.

- **Spend as much time as you can, naked.** This reacquaints you with your body and puts you in touch with your sexual self.

- **Devote an hour a week to loving your body.** If pampering isn't you, start exercising or go to a massage therapist or reflexologist. Anything that gets you back in touch with that thing you need for sex –your body.

'If you're one of those people who can't even look in the mirror naked, you need to get used to it. Maybe you need to start with underwear. Maybe you need to start with a Parka, and work down from there. The point is...you're going to have to get comfortable in your own skin.'
DR PHIL MCGRAW, writing in *O Magazine*

Defining idea...

207

How did
it go?

Q   I need to lose weight, but I just can't. What'll make me succeed?

A   *If you were thinner, how would you behave? What would you be doing?
Exercising, eating healthily, buying nice clothes? OK. How can you start
doing that tomorrow? The mistake most would-be slimmers make is to think
in abstract rather than concrete terms and be too ambitious. You can start
exercising tomorrow, but it's highly unlikely you'll start jogging round the
park four days a week, which is probably the unrealistic goal you've set
yourself. It's also highly unlikely you're going to give up chocolate and
crisps overnight, but you could aim to eat fruit or vegetables at every meal.
You could buy yourself one nice item of clothing, even if it's in a bigger size
– it will make you feel better about yourself. Build up until you're following
the sort of lifestyle that will mean you reach your goals.*

**Q   I find my partner less attractive since he got fat. He keeps saying
he'll do something about it, but his attempts last two days max.
Am I being unreasonable?**

A   *Your attitude is just the sort that won't help. Research studies have shown
that it takes people many attempts to succeed at reaching a weight goal,
but if they keep persevering, they'll get there. One of the factors that helps
them is the unwavering, non-judgemental support of family. That's you.*

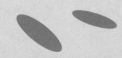

48

Dressed to kill

Whether it's fancy dress or a formal affair, what should you wear?

There is nothing worse than arriving at an event and realising that you have chosen completely the wrong outfit.

I think it is easier for women to get it wrong than men, because a man can bluff his way through most situations in a suit and tie: if you feel overdressed you simply remove the jacket and tie and you instantly look less formal. However, if a woman turns up in a little black dress accessorised with gorgeous jewels and everyone else has shown up in jeans, then it takes a great deal of composure to carry off the outfit without embarrassment. Of course, the first thing to do would be remove some of the glitter, but you are still going to stand out.

If you have received an invitation in the post, then the chances are that the dress code will be indicated on the card. Black tie means formal dress. Here's a note for men – don't try out a tie or waistcoat that features cartoon characters or comedy motifs. It may have seemed funny when you looked at it in the shop, but you'll probably regret wearing it when everyone else in the room has adhered to the traditional black tuxedo, white dress shirt and black bow tie. Not only that but you may well embarrass your date. Unless you are tall and slim, don't do a Bogart in

Here's an idea for you...

For women: when choosing a dress for a ball, wedding or party, pick a style that suits your build. If you are short or have a full figure, you might consider something 'empire line', which, with the seam just under the bust, means that the flowing fabric below is complementary to your shape. If you are tall and slim then a long, form-fitting dress can look stunning. Chubby arms look best in long loose sleeves; if you are quite bony, opt for fitted three-quarter length sleeves.

Casablanca and wear a white jacket; black is always more flattering on most men. And here's a note for women. Check with one or two friends or female members of your family to find out what they are going to wear so that you can gauge the style of your outfit accordingly. I'm not saying that you shouldn't be able to wear what you like, within reason, but you will be more comfortable if you fit in with others.

It is particularly important at weddings that men stick to the style that has been indicated and that women do not wear anything that will detract or take the focus away from the bride. You may think this seems a little boring, but you must bear in mind that you are probably going to be photographed with the couple. You do not want the bride and groom to be disappointed with their wedding album just because your outfit stands out in every picture.

The most important thing about following any dress code is that you feel happy and confident in what you are wearing. Don't vamp it up in your style of dress, if that's not the kind of person that you are. And don't think that you can rely on a couple of glasses to give you Dutch courage. Being tipsy and unhappy with how you look is twice as bad as being sober and unsure.

FANCY DRESS

These parties can be a tremendous success, with the photos passed around for months after the event, or they can be a damp squib if people don't join in. So if you are going to ask people to dress up, make sure that everyone who is invited knows about it – and make sure they know that coming in 'normal' party clothes is unacceptable. There is nothing worse than donning a bunny outfit and walking into a room – or garden in the case of Bridget Jones – when most of the other people haven't 'turned out'. As a guest, the best way to avoid this happening is to go and hire outfits with a group of friends so that you know there'll be safety in numbers.

If you are going to throw a fancy dress party it makes it a simpler prospect for people to decide what to wear if you give the evening a theme. Heroes and Villains is always a good one and Nursery Rhymes provides plenty of scope if there are going to be children at the party too.

Whatever the choice, party gear or fancy dress, plan your outfit well in advance to avoid last minute panics and the possibility that 'you don't have anything to wear'!

'Clothes make the man. Naked people have little or no influence on society.'
MARK TWAIN

'Clothes and manners do not make the man; but when he is made, they greatly improve his appearance.'
ARTHUR ASHE

Defining idea...

Defining idea...

How did it go?

Q **I know that I have to be smart but I am confused about the difference between black tie and white tie. Can you straighten this out?**

A *Black tie means that you are expected to wear a tuxedo whereas white tie indicates that the man should wear a tail coat (which is one step up from a dinner jacket in the formal stakes) and a white tie. 'White tie' is more formal.*

Q **Right, that's me sorted – but what about my date?**

A *White tie for ladies indicates that they should consider wearing something long and glamorous; it's not appropriate to wear a short dress to something where white tie is specified. Black tie simply means a smart look – it could be a two-piece outfit like an evening trouser suit or a smart, cocktail-type dress.*

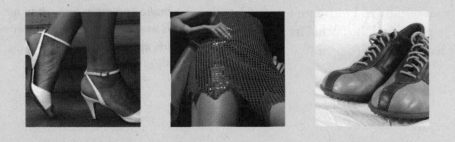

49

Clever hair care

Simple tricks to turn a bad hair day good, plus hairdos to knock years off you.

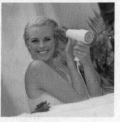

Genetics, weather, hormones, diet and hair products (too many, not enough or the wrong type) can all take their toll. If you're frizzy, flat or frumpy, you need some professional help.

Our experts have done the legwork for you, so try these invaluable solutions to everyday hair headaches.

BOOK THAT TRIM

A regular trim – every six to eight weeks – really is the best way to keep your hair in tip-top condition. Each hair on your head grows at its own pace, so within weeks they can look uneven and scraggly. Split ends happen when the individual layers of hair shafts separate due to chemicals, weather or too much heat from styling. You can help to seal split ends by using a leave-in conditioner, but the effect will only be

Here's an idea for you...

Put your hair in a high ponytail and you'll look years younger. It will help lift your face. A fringe can knock years off you too, plus it can emphasise your cheekbones. And highlights around your face are anti-ageing as they lighten and brighten your complexion.

temporary. Your hair grows between a third and half an inch per month, so you'll recover the length again in no time. A trim will make your hair look thicker, healthier and glossier.

THE BEST BLOW-DRY

■ Blot wet hair first with a towel. If your hair is fine, only condition the ends because if you put it on the roots you'll make it lank. Spray some gel onto the roots and spread it evenly by rubbing with your fingers. To control frizz, use a small dollop of smoothing balm rather than gel, which can make hair drier.

■ For added volume, use a handful of mousse about the size of a golf ball. Also, try wrapping the top layers of your hair around two large Velcro rollers when you're hair is 95% dry and then finish blow-drying.

■ Wait until your hair is quite dry before you blow-dry it and you'll do less damage; hair can lose up to 30% of its moisture when blow-dried.

■ Clip your hair up into sections. Start with the hair at the back of your head first, then the side sections. Pull each section taut with a large round brush and dry from the root to the tip. Use the nozzle to tuck the ends under or to lift hair from the roots for volume.

■ After drying each section, give it a blast of cold air to help 'set' the hair.

■ When you hair is totally dry, part it. Now's the time to add a bit of serum to coarse, long or curly hair. Otherwise, wait until the hair is cool then spritz your hands with hairspray and rub it over your hair.

TIPS FOR CURLY OR FRIZZY HAIR

Frizz is the result of too much heat, sun or chemicals used to bleach, colour, straighten or curl your hair.

- Choose conditioners with panthenol and silicone, which make the cuticle lie flat and make hair look smoother and sleeker.
- If you have naturally wiry or wispy hair, always use conditioner after shampooing and also invest in a deep-conditioning product. Also, wash your hair thoroughly to get rid of traces of shampoo and conditioner; otherwise it'll look lank. You'll know when you've washed away the last of the residue because when you run your hand through your hair, it should feel squeaky-clean.
- Never use too much conditioner even if your hair is thick. The right size for shoulder length hair is that of an almond, less if it's shorter.
- Blot hair with a towel to absorb excess moisture. A wide-toothed comb can detangle curly hair without tearing it and help to eliminate frizz. Anything else can break or tear your hair, leaving it with split ends.
- Apply a protective product before you blow-dry to prevent hair from dehydrating and then use a diffuser and your fingers to gently blow-dry. Avoid brushes or combs, as they'll just make your hair frizz. After drying, rub a few drops of serum into the palms of your hands then smooth it over your hair to calm wayward strands and seal in moisture.

'Hair style is the final tip-off whether or not a woman really knows herself.'
HUBERT DE GIVENCHY

Defining idea...

'I'm not offended by all the dumb-blonde jokes because I know that I'm not dumb. I also know I'm not blonde.'
DOLLY PARTON

Defining idea...

How did it go?

Q   I have really fine hair. Is there anything I can do to thicken it up?

A   Unfortunately, you drew the short straw. There's nothing you can do to permanently thicken fine hair. It's genetic, just like colour, texture, curliness and straightness. Do make sure you're eating plenty of protein-rich foods though, such as meat, fish, tofu and dairy products, as these will help to build strong hair. The best way to thicken hair is through products: wash your hair with volumising shampoo, coat it with a leave-in conditioner to bulk it up and use gels and mousses to add body. Also, waves and curls always have more body than straight hair, so play around with different styles and rollers. And colouring your hair or adding highlights can add texture that will give the impression of thickness. Finally, get it cut regularly, as split ends make hair look finer and more damaged.

Q   How can I make a lovely blow-dry last?

A   Before you get into the shower, clip your hair up in a high bun and wear a shower cap; whatever you feel about shower caps they're great for keeping the heat in, which will help lift the roots. Wait until the hair – and you – are completely dry before unclipping it. And avoid getting it wet at all costs, as moisture will cause it to kink or curl, so never go out without an umbrella or even a rain bonnet. (I know, but it does the trick.)

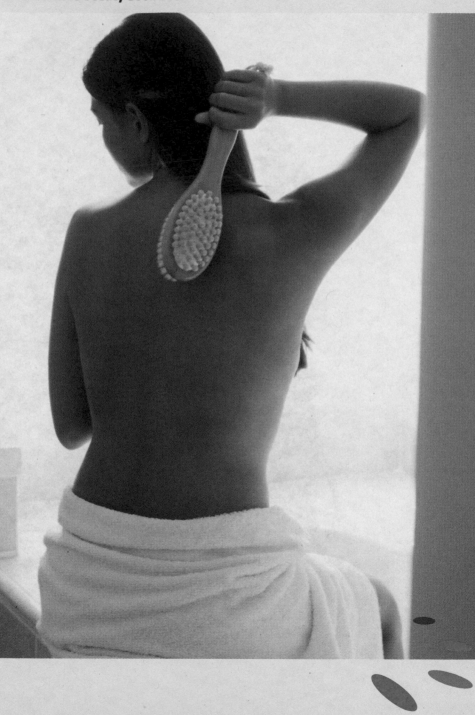

50

Let's face facts

Skin is your body's biggest organ. It mirrors your inner health and, unlike your other organs, the world gets to look at it.

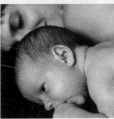

Pale, blotchy skin says you're not looking after yourself in some respect. You can do much to improve it though from both the outside and inside. It's simply a question of finding the right products for you, then actually using them!

BEFORE WE START

Sunshine – don't we just love it? There are some real health benefits to be had from being in sunshine, but like everything you can have too much of a good thing. The trouble is, sunshine is dehydrating, as hot sun will increase the evaporation of water from the surface of the skin. You need plenty of antioxidants or agents that protect us against harmful environmental factors. These can be found in, you guessed it, fruit and vegetables. Obviously, plenty of water is the order of the day too – at least

Here's an idea for you...

Treat yourself to a facial massage. They're wonderful for the circulation – the Aveda salons (www.aveda.com) are great for this and although they tend to be hellishly expensive, they're well worth the investment in my opinion. Alternatively do it yourself with a home massage – Neal's Yard (www.nealsyardremedies.com) do some great oils, especially the rose face oils. A number of websites give advice on this: Google 'facial massage' and enjoy.

2 litres (3.5 pints) of the stuff. And knock off the cigarettes and the alcohol! You know it is bad for you and it's really not helping your body's detoxification pathways (your liver in particular). One last nag, remember to incorporate lots of essential fatty acids in your diet as your skin needs to be well oiled, so include lots of nuts, seeds and oily fish in your diet.

ROUTINE, ROUTINE!

I remember friends laughing at me at university for using expensive products on my skin. There's nothing wrong with soap and water they cried. The decades take a poor view of soap and water, in my opinion. I've always used expensive products, right from when my mum set me up with my first skincare regime when I was about thirteen. Of course, you don't have to spend a fortune on skincare, and expensive doesn't always equal good, but getting into a routine is vital. I found that my expensive products made me want to use them and their value was reflected in my skin.

The second thing I learnt very early on in my life was to always take your make-up off, however late you get to bed! When I was fifteen, my best friend Helena stayed over after a party. At four in the morning, there she was carefully taking off all her make-up. She had beautiful clear skin whereas I, already in bed with a smudged party face, had a face like a pizza. From that moment on, regardless of the time, I've always properly cleansed my face.

The most important thing you can do to perk your skin up is to exfoliate. Exfoliation isn't something you need to do every day – once a week should be fine. As we get older, we really need to make sure we're exfoliating on a really regular basis otherwise if we don't clear out the dead cells, wrinkles can look deeper. Older skin too needs a gentler touch when it comes to exfoliation – no pulling and rubbing or harsh products like creams based on fruit acids. Fresh (www.fresh.com) has a really wonderful facial scrub that is moisturising at the same time. Alternatively, make your own exfoliator with 2 teaspoons of fine oatmeal and 2 teaspoons of ground almonds with some rose water to blend. Rub it in small circular motions over your skin, then rinse off.

'You can have anything you want – if you want it badly enough. You can be anything you want to be, do anything you set out to accomplish, if you hold to that desire with singleness of purpose.'
WILLIAM ADAMS (so if you want beautiful skin, start looking after it!)

Defining idea...

How did
it go?

Q   **My skin really looks dull. What can I do for an instant pick-me-up?**

A   *Treat yourself to a mask. There are some brilliant ones on the market, but the ones that I love at the moment are REN's Multi-Mineral Detox Facial Mask and REN's Jirgolulan Cell Energising Facial Mask (both available from www.beautyexpert.co.uk).*

Q   **I've tried everything and my skin still looks dull and flat. Any suggestions?**

A   *It might be worth investing in a facial. I really like the Clarins' facials as they're usually not the most expensive one yet you still come out with skin that looks like its been on holiday. The extra boost you get from professional help can often prompt you to look after your skin more carefully yourself.*

Q   **With all this talk about my face, what about my body?**

A   *A cheap way to exfoliate your skin is to use sea salt as a scrub. Scrub your body all over (avoiding the really sensitive areas) and rinse, if you can stand it, in cold water to give your skin a real tingle.*

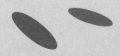

51

Dieting danger

Disordered eating is frightening, confusing and poses severe health risks. While the causes are complex and not fully understood, everyone should be aware of the danger signs of eating habits that are getting out of control.

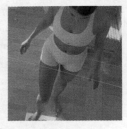

Contrary to popular belief, eating disorders are not a modern illness — they have been going on for centuries. What is true, is that they now seem to be on the increase.

Much disordered eating is kept secret until it becomes patently obvious that there's a problem, so it is hard to put any real figures on how many sufferers there really are. More and more people are coming forward for help and treatment for themselves or their friends and family members.

Eating disorders are difficult to understand, whether you're a sufferer or watching someone else suffer, but I think it is especially hard on the latter group. Why does someone who has starved themselves still insist they're fat? What is going on in the mind of someone who looks perfectly gorgeous yet steals away to the bathroom a few times a week to vomit? How can they be ashamed of what they've eaten and afraid to gain weight when they are obviously thin?

Here's an idea for you... **Get yourself along to a self-help group. Talking to others who have experienced the same issues and problems and can offer support and understanding without blaming you or making you feel guilty, can be a real help.**

Some experts think there is a link between dieting and developing eating disorders, especially bulimia. The theory goes that dieting makes you hungry, which makes you binge, which then makes you feel guilty. In susceptible people, a purge (vomiting or using laxatives), helps to deal with the guilt and 'remove' the calories.

There are millions of us who diet without developing these kinds of illnesses. What has been discovered is that people who have eating disorders also share certain personality traits – they are perfectionists, who are eager to please, yet who have low self-esteem. When these factors are combined with family troubles (divorce, bereavement) or indeed certain family attitudes to weight and food, the spiral into illness can be quick. Ultimately, eating disorders are usually about control.

Treatment is available, but success is dependent on the individual accepting help. Even then, there are a proportion of people who will continue to obsess about weight and food for the rest of their lives. Anorexics will usually be referred to a specialist psychiatrist who is experienced in eating disorders, which may be enough to get attitudes to food and eating back to somewhere approaching healthy. However, some anorexics will be hospitalised because of the lack of fluids and nutrients in their bodies, which is even more distressing, not only for the carers, but for the sufferer themselves as they feel themselves losing what little control they have in their lives. For bulimics, anti-depressants have been found to help reduce bingeing, but psychological treatment is essential too.

Check whether your own eating habits and attitudes, or those of a friend or family member, could indicate signs of disordered eating. If you're concerned, see your doctor, contact a self-help group or check The Eating Disorders Association at www.edauk.com.

The following is not an exhaustive list, but some common indications that issues exist or are beginning to develop include:

- Not eating in front of others, claiming to have just eaten or having prepared a meal for others.

- Being secretive around food.

- A strong fear of gaining weight, although you have an acceptable weight or are even underweight.

- Distorted body image – believing you're fat when you're at an acceptable weight or underweight.

'It's important to remember that eating disorders are very complex conditions and are not about dieting going too far. The vast majority of people who diet don't have eating disorders.'
LYNDEL COSTAIN, *Diet Trials: How to Succeed at Dieting*

Defining idea...

225

- Recurrent bingeing – eating too much in a short space of time, i.e. within a few hours.

- Shame and guilt after eating leading to using laxatives, or making yourself vomit.

- Obsession with exercise – working out several times a day for a couple of hours at a time.

- Judging yourself solely on looks.

- Ritualistic eating habits such as cutting food into tiny pieces.

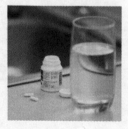 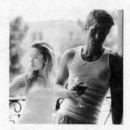 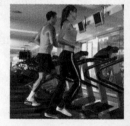

Q **I think about food all the time, especially about what I've just eaten and what I'll eat next. I don't have a problem, do I?**

How did it go?

A *Maybe not, but it doesn't sound as though your relationship with food is all that healthy either. Sorry to sound nannyish, but you could probably use some professional support, via a nutritionist or friendly doctor.*

Q **I have a friend who has dieted as long as I've known her. I'm sure she's anorexic but she gets really angry if I try to talk to her about it. What can I do?**

A *Of course you want to help, but often this will be perceived as criticism or pressure which will only make things worse. All you can do is be there, listen, love and support. Once your friend has recognised she has a problem, you can lend practical support in finding help, going along to medical appointments and so on.*

Q **I binge, but don't vomit or use laxatives. So I'm OK, aren't I?**

A *Many binge eaters eat to escape their emotions, but then feel that food makes them out of control. If you binge but don't purge, you may well also be very overweight. Medical help is essential to get you out of this behaviour. Pluck up the courage to ask for it. You won't regret it.*

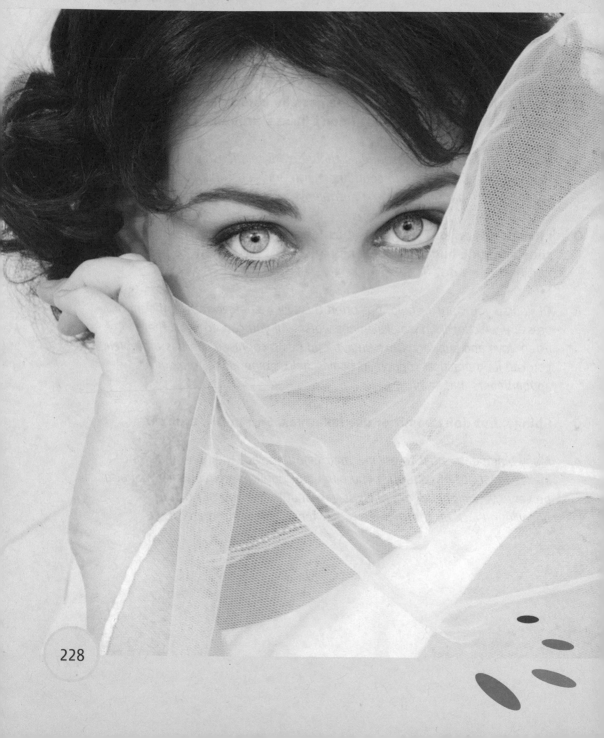

228

52

Enhance your eyes

They're said to be the windows to the soul, the first thing people notice and capable of disarming a man at 100 paces. But what if your eyes are more Mole Man than Bette Davis?

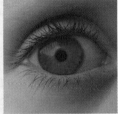

According to anthropologists, the most attractive women's faces are 'child-like', with smooth skin, a peaches-and-cream complexion, a small nose and big eyes with long Bambi lashes.

These are all good reasons to take care of your eyes. Easy-peasy eye care includes taking off your eye make-up every night, keeping dirty hankies or fingers away from them and patting instead of rubbing the skin surrounding them. Make sure you get lots of sleep, drink gallons of water, apply a regular dab of eye cream and treat yourself to the odd cucumber or teabag session.

As for making them bigger and veiled in long, thick, fluttery eyelashes, you'll need a few good tools and clever make-up techniques.

Here's an idea for you...

Bring out the colour of your eyes using contrasts. Pinks, mauves and greys look great on blue eyes. Or use really dark colours for stunning contrasts. Avoid pinks if your eyes are red and tired; stick to neutrals or ivories instead. Remember: blend, blend, blend.

Try these:

- Start with your eyebrows and pluck any stray hairs with a pair of tweezers.
- Apply a pale or neutral colour over the upper eyelid, blending over the outer edges, to give a good matt base on which you can blend and build darker and stronger colours. Even a dab of foundation can create a great base for colour and cover any redness or blotchiness.
- Apply a brown or grey eyeshadow, from the middle to the outer edge of the eye. Start with a tiny bit of colour and add more layers, blending as you go.
- Brush a thin line of a darker shade along the upper lid. Add a little shading under the eye, too, at the outer edge.
- Using white pencil along the lower inner socket of your eyes can make them more striking. Or dot a tiny spot of white shadow in the inner corners of your eyes to make them look wider apart.
- If your eyes are small, remember that you'll make them look even smaller by using eyeshadow or eyeliner around the entire eye as this will effectively close them up.
- False eyelashes can really open up the eyes so don't be afraid of them. Try a few individual lashes on the outer corner of the eye, then add a few shorter ones, and alternate between the two as you work towards the middle of the eye.
- Invest in eyelash curlers, which really help to open your eyes. They're easier to use than they look, too. Just hold them so that your upper lashes lie between the two rims, then squeeze and roll upwards.

- Eyeshadow spillage? Before you start, pop a layer of translucent loose powder underneath each eye to catch any of the eyeshadow that falls on your cheeks. You can then simply brush it away and you don't have to reapply foundation.

> '*Cosmetics is a boon to every woman, but a girl's best beauty aid is still a near-sighted man.*'
> YOKO ONO

Defining idea...

- Stick to black mascara for drama, brown if you're very blonde, or try the 'no make-up' look, which is also more flattering against older skins.
- Some make-up artists recommend you put mascara on the top lashes only and leave the bottom ones bare – it makes you look brighter and less tired.
- Don't dismiss coloured mascara. Try navy blue (not electric blue) to make the whites of your eyes look whiter, or plum, which can look great on blondes.
- Avoid putting powder underneath your eyes, as when it 'cakes' it shows up every crease and fine line and can be very ageing.
- How many layers of mascara? Ideally two for maximum drama, but don't let it dry between layers or it may cake and flake.
- Invest in eyedrops, a great way to put a sparkle in your eye.

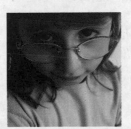

How did it go?

Q **My eyes aren't particularly small, but they are deep set. How can I make them more noticeable?**

A *Start by applying a pale eyeshadow or even a concealer over your entire eyelid. This will immediately lighten and 'brighten' your eyelid and effectively bring your eyes 'forward'. Try using a darker colour along the lashline to help elongate the eye, blending from the centre of the eye to the outer corner. You can define your eyes further by slicking on lots of mascara.*

Q **My eyes are dark brown so should I avoid coloured eyeshadows?**

A *There are no rules these days, so play around with some colours and just see what works. Pale pinks or lilacs can look fantastic. Natural tones do look great with dark eyes, though – look for browns, blacks, peachy colours or almond shades. To dress up your make-up for evenings, make the contrast between dark shades and creams even more dramatic.*

Q **What's the best way to perk up droopy lids?**

A *To lift them, measure about a third of the way in from the outer corner of the eyelid then draw a line of mid-colour shadow from the lash line to the browbone. Build up the colour using a brush and blend it in from the browbone to the inner corner of your eyelid. Then simply add a bit of pale eyeshadow in the corner of the eye to open it up more.*

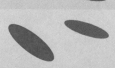

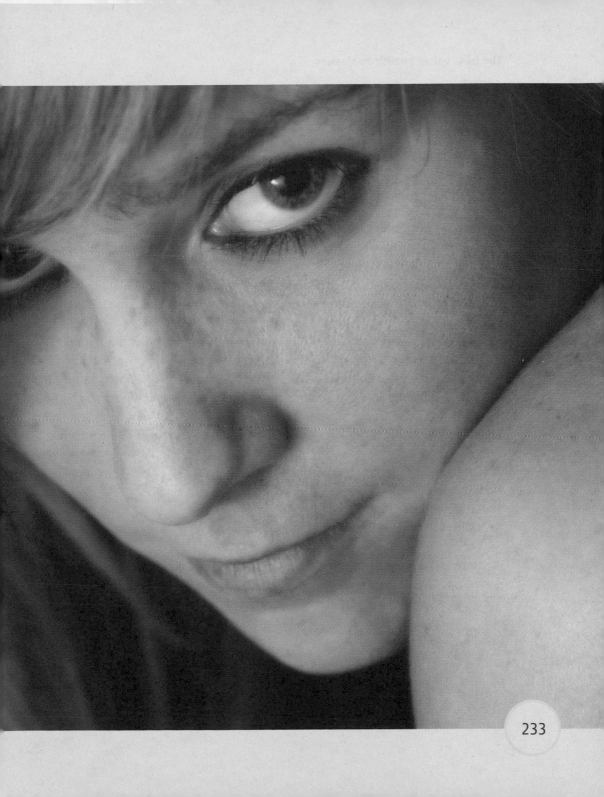

The end...

Or is it a new beginning? We hope that the ideas in this book will have inspired you to try some new things to be your beautiful best. You've discovered that a handful of carefully chosen and cleverly applied beauty products along with a few dietary changes and a sackful of self-confidence can go a long way. Hopefully the tips you read here will have you turning heads every time you walk down the street.

So why not let *us* know all about it? Tell us how you got on. What did it for you – what really made you stop traffic? Maybe you've got some tips of your own you want to share (see next page if so). And if you liked this book you may find we have even more brilliant ideas that could change other areas of your life for the better.

You'll find the Infinite Ideas crew waiting for you online at www.infideas.com.

Or if you prefer to write, then send your letters to:
The best value BEAUTY book ever
The Infinite Ideas Company Ltd
36 St Giles, Oxford OX1 3LD, United Kingdom

We want to know what you think, because we're all working on making our lives better too. Give us your feedback and you could win a copy of another *52 Brilliant Ideas* book of your choice. Or maybe get a crack at writing your own.

Good luck. Be brilliant.

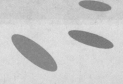

Offer one

CASH IN YOUR IDEAS

We hope you enjoy this book. We hope it inspires, amuses, educates and entertains you. But we don't assume that you're a novice, or that this is the first book that you've bought on the subject. You've got ideas of your own. Maybe our author has missed an idea that you use successfully. If so, why not send it to yourauthormissedatrick@infideas.com, and if we like it we'll post it on our bulletin board. Better still, if your idea makes it into print we'll send you four books of your choice or the cash equivalent. You'll be fully credited so that everyone knows you've had another Brilliant Idea.

Offer two

HOW COULD YOU REFUSE?

Amazing discounts on bulk quantities of Infinite Ideas books are available to corporations, professional associations and other organisations.

For details call us on:
+44 (0)1865 514888
Fax: +44 (0)1865 514777
or e-mail: info@infideas.com

Where it's at...

brilliant ideas

The Best Value Ever Series is published by Infinite Ideas, publishers of the acclaimed **52 Brilliant Ideas** series and a range of other titles which are all life-enhancing and entertaining. If you found this book of interest, you may want to take advantage of this special offer. Choose any two books from the selection below and you'll get one of them free of charge*. See p. 242 for prices and details on how to place your order.

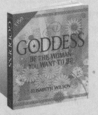

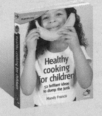

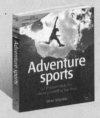

Goddess
Be the woman YOU want to be Edited by Elisabeth Wilson
BUMPER BOOK – CONTAINS 149 IDEAS!

Healthy cooking for Children
52 brilliant ideas to dump the junk
By Mandy Francis

Adventure sports
52 brilliant ideas for taking yourself to the limit
By Steve Shipside

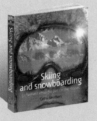

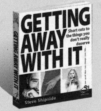

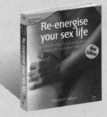

Skiing and snowboarding
52 brilliant ideas for fun on the slopes
By Cathy Struthers

Getting away with it
Shortcuts to the things you don't really deserve
Compiled by Steve Shipside

Re-energise your sex life (2nd edition)
52 brilliant ideas to put the zing back into your lovemaking
By Elisabeth Wilson

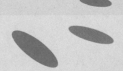

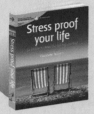

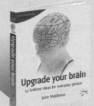

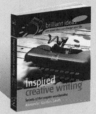

Stress proof your life
52 brilliant ideas for taking control
By Elisabeth Wilson

Upgrade your brain
52 brilliant ideas for everyday genius
By John Middleton

Inspired creative writing
Secrets of the master wordsmiths
By Alexander Gordon Smith

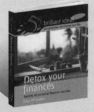

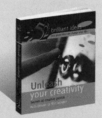

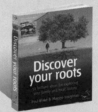

Detox your finances
Secrets of personal finance success
By John Middleton

Unleash your creativity
Secrets of creative genius
By Rob Bevan &
Tim Wright

Discover your roots
52 brilliant ideas for exploring your family & local history
By Paul Blake &
Maggie Loughran

For more detailed information on these books and others published by Infinite Ideas please visit www.infideas.com

The best value beauty book ever

Choose any two titles from below and receive the cheapest one free.

Qty	Title	RRP
	Goddess	£18.99
	Healthy cooking for children	£12.99
	Adventure sports	£12.99
	Skiing and snowboarding	£12.99
	Getting away with it	£6.99
	Re-energise your sex life (2ND EDITION)	£12.99
	Stress proof your life	£12.99
	Upgrade your brain	£12.99
	Inspired creative writing	£12.99
	Unleash your creativity	£12.99
	Detox your finances	£12.99
	Discover your roots	£12.99
	Subtract lowest priced book if ordering two titles	
	Add £2.75 postage per delivery address	
	Final TOTAL	

Name: ....

Delivery address: ....

....

....

....

E-mail:..Tel (in case of problems): ....

By post Fill in all relevant details, cut out or photocopy this page and send along with a cheque made payable to Infinite Ideas. Send to: Re-energise Offer, Infinite Ideas, 36 St Giles, Oxford OX1 3LD, UK.

Credit card orders over the telephone Call +44 (0) 1865 514 888. Lines are open 9am to 5pm Monday to Friday. Just mention the promotion code 'BVAD06.'

Please note that no payment will be processed until your order has been dispatched. Goods are dispatched through Royal Mail within 14 working days, when in stock. We never forward personal details on to third parties or bombard you with junk mail. This offer is valid for UK and RoI residents only. Any questions or comments please contact us on 01865 514 888 or email info@infideas.com.

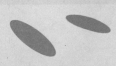